To Our Mastermind Family,

Gratitude and appreciation are key elements to living a life of fulfillment. Personally, I am so grateful for this partnership with Mastermind Toys, especially to its Founders, my cousins Jon and Andy Levy. Growing up as kids together on the shores of Lake Simcoe, we would all gather by the frigid water on the May 24th weekend to take the annual Uncle Ed's Polar Bear dip. We cheered each other on as we took turns taking that shocking plunge. For years this communal dunk became a source of excitement, love and inclusiveness.

Since our son Jacob's devastating diagnosis 19 years ago, Mastermind Toys has been an integral part of the momentum and success of our charity Jacob's Ladder. Although a different type of plunge, the Mastermind Family has been with us every step of the way. Due to their generosity, loyalty and devotion, we have been able to climb to new heights with each passing year. Their support gave us strength.

Community involvement makes us all better, stronger and kinder. Mastermind Toys is equally appreciative for your on going loyalty. With this in mind, this book is for YOU. Hopefully it will help you through your own hardships and help turn your challenges into triumphs.

This special edition of *Without One Word Spoken* is a gift from our hearts to yours. Let's take that plunge together.

Love, Ellen

Without One Word Spoken isn't just the compelling story of a child's miraculous life. It's also a mother's how-to of survival and joy.

– Craig Offman, *The Globe and Mail* Newspaper

■

What can a child who can't walk, talk, move or see teach us about life? As it turns out, everything. Supremely uplifting, at times heart-breaking, these 18 everyday lessons carefully crafted from years of caring for a child with a debilitating illness will change your life.

– Catherine Phillips, *Toronto Star*

■

Wow! Readers are in for a heart-to-heart story told by the ever-inspiring Ellen Schwartz who will take you on a journey of love, laughter and tears with life lessons that will resonate with everyone. I couldn't put it down. Thank you Jacob for being you—a different kind of perfect!

– Susan Minuk, Freelance Writer and Journalist

When Ellen shared this manuscript with me, little did I know I would be getting life-changing advice. Whether it is hugging my family a little bit tighter (20 seconds to be exact), knowing instinctively how to give vs asking how can I help or memorizing every part of a moment. ... This is a page turning book that makes you want to complete it and then read it again and again. I took so many notes because I just wanted to be sure I remembered all the sage advice. Jacob was put on this planet for a reason and I am so grateful to have had the opportunity to learn all that he can teach us.

– Carolyn Everson, mom of twin girls,
Vice President of Global Marketing Solutions, Facebook

Without One Word Spoken

18 Life Lessons from Jacob

Ellen Schwartz

Brilliant
Idea Books

Library and Archives Canada Cataloguing in Publication

Schwartz, Ellen (Ellen A.)

  Without one word spoken : 18 life lessons from Jacob / Ellen Schwartz.

ISBN 978-0-9938387-5-0 (paperback)

    1. Schwartz, Jacob, 1997- —Health. 2. Canavan disease—
Patients—Canada—Biography. 3. Canavan disease—Patients—Family
relationships—Canada. I. Title.

RJ496.C42S395 2016   618.92'830092   C2016-905348-2

ISBN 978-0-9938387-5-0
e-book ISBN 978-0-9938387-7-4

Publisher: Brilliant Idea Books
Edited by: Randi Chapnik Myers
Proofread by: Catherine Leek of Green Onion Publishing
Front Cover Designed by: Cynthia Cake of WeMakeBooks.ca
Text Design, Layout and Print Production by: Beth Crane of WeMakeBooks.ca

Printed and bound in Canada

For Jeff, Bevvy, Ben and Jake.

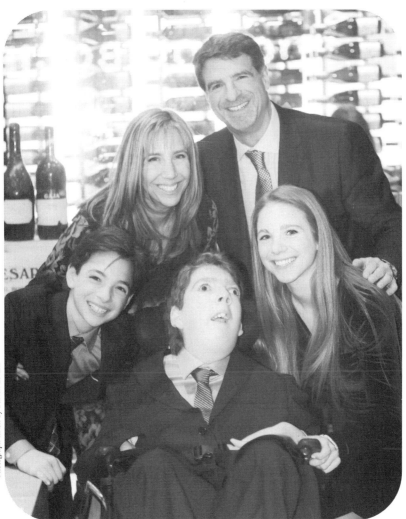

TABLE OF CONTENTS

Believe in Miracles

When you wake up every day
Please don't throw your dreams away
Hold them close to your heart
Cause we're all a part
Of the ordinary miracle

— Sarah McLachlan

Do you believe in miracles? I do, and here's why.

Like all girls, I had dreams and aspirations. When I was really young, I told everyone I wanted to be a famous singer or actress because that seemed like the glamorous choice. Later, I pretended I wanted to be a doctor or lawyer like most of my friends because that seemed like the intelligent choice. The truth was, though, that my dream was to be Somebody's Mom. I couldn't wait for the day when I could hold and cuddle that newborn child of mine. That day finally arrived when I was 30 years old.

I embraced every kick and twist from the baby growing inside of me. I loved every minute of those nine months. When we met

Jacob William Schwartz, our first child, his strapping healthy nine pounds meant I had arrived, too.

Like all new parents, we were equally overwhelmed by joy and fear. We went to prenatal classes to help us prepare for anything and everything. For months, I had been immersed in articles, books and videos about parenthood. There was nothing that my husband, Jeff, and I couldn't handle together. We were a team, and now a healthy threesome, setting out to write the next chapter of our dream.

And then, everything changed.

All of the books stated that Jacob's eyes would follow me, the mother. I was the center of my child's world, the one who bore him, the one who held his milk. His eyes never followed.

All of the books stated that in a few weeks, he would start to raise his head. We waited and waited. Whenever Jacob tried to lift his head, it just flopped back down.

He started crying, and crying, and crying. All of the books stated that colic was a normal part of child development, but the crying didn't stop.

Something was wrong with Jacob.

We were lucky to have a pediatrician who was on the ball. He sent us down to the Hospital for Sick Children in Toronto for a plethora of tests. Jeff and I hugged our two-month-old as doctors and nurses poked and prodded him, hunting for answers.

Why wasn't Jacob meeting the simplest of milestones? What was wrong with Jacob?

Most newborns spend their days cuddled up in a warm blanket in their bassinet or nestled in the loving arms of doting family members. Jacob spent his first months in hospital waiting rooms or lying naked on procedure beds not knowing what was coming next. How could our baby understand what was happening to him when we, his parents, had no clue?

When Jacob was just four months old, the hospital called. It was the metabolic and genetics team.

"We have good news and bad news." Being the eternal optimist, I asked for the good news first. "The good news is we know what is wrong with Jacob. The bad news is, it isn't very good news."

Soon, we were sitting in a hospital room, absorbing Jacob's diagnosis and prognosis. Our eyes grew wide as we faced this devastating reality.

"Jacob has a rare, fatal, neurodegenerative illness that attacks the central nervous system. It is called Canavan Disease, a disease for which there is no known treatment or cure. Children with Canavan Disease cannot crawl, walk, sit or talk. Over time, they may suffer seizures, become paralyzed or blind, and have trouble swallowing. Death usually occurs before the age of four, although some children may survive into their teens."

In that instant, my dreams for a family life of fulfillment and bliss vanished. Hearing the words that our precious boy would likely never live past the age of four, we braced for a downward spiral. Surely, we were in for a life of sadness, sickness and challenges so huge they'd be too much to handle. Our baby had his whole life ahead and now it felt like a life sentence. In fact, over the years, I have been reminded many times by doctors and therapists, "Remember, Ellen, Jacob is on borrowed time."

Well, it's a good thing I am terrible at returning things because somehow, some way, the clock is still ticking. And somehow, we found a way to find joy. Because of Jacob's journey, we have learned lessons about life, about living it in a conscious way, where we have choices about our own actions and perspectives. Somehow, in the depths of life's darkness, a miracle happened.

These lessons came from years of caring for a child with a debilitating illness. Canavan Disease robbed Jacob of almost every possible physical and mental ability. The doctors were partially right. Our child can't walk, talk, move or see. He is fed by a tube through his stomach. Because he has a hard time managing his own secretions, his body often needs suctioning. He requires one-on-one attention at all times.

At first, when the doctors delivered the terrible news, we were sure that our lives were over. We were devastated, heartbroken and completely discouraged. We needed to try something, anything, to help Jacob, and to help ourselves.

There was one chance. We enrolled him in a ground-breaking experimental gene replacement trial at Yale University in New Haven, Connecticut. It was a risky procedure, but it also gave us a shred of hope. And it turned out to be the "Aha!" moment we desperately needed in order to go on.

The results were not what we hoped for. Complications from the trial caused Jacob to experience a seizure that lasted an hour and a half. He spent months lying in a hospital room fighting meningitis and hydrocephalus, his little head wrapped in bandages. Our baby underwent seven operations in just two months. To be perfectly honest, this time in our lives is a bit of a blur to me now. Is it my mind protecting my heart from the pain? It could be. Is it the repetition of sleepless nights causing a mental fog that clogged up my memory? It could be that as well. All I know is that it was a time when I felt completely vulnerable, hopeless, helpless and scared. Not a good combination of emotions.

The "Aha!" moment came during this time. It was when Jeff was lying on his back in the hospital bed with little Jacob stretched out on his daddy's stomach. He was resting inside the safety net of those strong arms wrapped around him, finally sleeping after hours of screaming. Jeff wouldn't move for fear of waking Jacob, of risking his feeling of peace. It was at that moment when the miracle appeared.

If we could help it, we decided, our child would never experience pain ever again. While we couldn't save Jacob from the disease he was born with, we could accept it and make his life as comfortable and as peaceful as possible. Once we stopped trying to cure Jacob, our lives changed again—this time, for the better. Now, he was the one with the power to help cure us.

Interestingly, it wasn't until I came to grips with this new reality that I realized I had a choice: To accept the life sentence and give up on my dreams or to open up to the possibility of letting new dreams unfold.

As I wrote in my recent book *Lessons from Jacob, A Disabled Son Teaches His Mother About Courage, Hope and The Joy of Living Each*

Day to the Fullest, living with someone who has a life threatening disease is beyond difficult. It can sometimes feel impossible. But in many ways, it is also a gift. It challenges your perspective on life, pushing you to think and act beyond the ordinary into the extraordinary. And that's what this book will help you do in your times of need.

The life lessons in *Without One Word Spoken* are based on the ripple effects of an extremely precious life—a life that could have been tragic and yet has somehow managed to fill so many lives with hope, joy and merit. These lessons are the result of the choices we make and the mindfulness of our thoughts and actions as we live each day.

For all of us, life is hard, ever changing and messy. What I know for sure is this: We only have control of one thing—our attitude—how we think and how we behave. Everything else that befalls us is waiting in the wings, a direct result of our own actions.

Let's examine the idea of attitude. While I could dwell on the past 19 years of sleepless nights, I choose instead to focus on Jacob's ability to wake up every day. That small blessing, that miracle, drives me to wake up physically, morally and mentally. And as the day unfolds, Jacob's outlook changes mine. His appreciation for the little things in life helps me to see how miraculous they are.

There are so many moments in each day that can get you down, that can drop your spirits or render you frustrated or anxious or angry if you let them. But your attitude in the face of challenge is your choice.

I know that if I am frustrated by misplacing my glasses or car keys, or at my wits' end about the disastrous state of my teenagers' bedrooms or annoyed that Jeff is late for dinner and it's sitting there getting cold, I have a choice. I can let these small upsets brew inside of me and let them fester into an unnecessary argument that ends up with two sides very unhappy. Or, I can realize that these are just small distractions that don't impact anything, other than my nerves.

All I have to do is look at Jacob and I am reminded that it has been one amazing day. I try so hard not to dwell on negativity because, when I do, it only makes the problem worse.

The fact is, we all have countless choices to make every day—everything from mundane ones such as whether to order dinner or make it from scratch to bigger ones like whether to leave a secure job to pursue a lifelong passion. Big or small, when it comes to choices, there really are only two options. You can learn from what each life lesson may be teaching you and move forward armed with new knowledge, or pity yourself for your misfortune and move in reverse, missing out on the lesson altogether.

The hard truth is that life can be tough and unfair, even tragic, but how we get through it is our choice. Whether you are a daughter, son, mother, father, sister or brother, you will face many unexpected turns, trials and tribulations and it will be how you choose to deal with each one that makes all the difference.

Think of a teeter-totter constantly moving up and down, up and down. Imagine if it was always in balance. What fun would that be?

Despite what you've been told, the key to life is not in finding balance in everything you do. Instead, it is in finding concrete ways to embrace the highs and to learn from the lows. It is in these two extremes that the fun, the growth and the blessings of life can be found.

This year Jacob turned 19. Nineteen!

That means that every day for almost the past two decades has been a blessing. And that's why I am sharing valuable life lessons that I have learned from each miraculous year of caring for him. Please use each of the following chapters to help guide you through your own struggles, step by step, whatever they might be. Feel free to flip to any chapter that might help you, and to use the strategies at the end of each one.

Do you believe in miracles yet? Read on. You will.

Celebrate Life, Whenever You Can

I welcome the sun
The clouds and rain
The wind that sweeps the sky clean and lets the sun shine again
This is the most magnificent life has ever been
Here is heaven and earth and the brilliant sky in between

Blessed is this life and I'm gonna celebrate being alive
Blessed is this life and I'm gonna celebrate being alive

– Brett Dennen, *Blessed*

Mornings are hard for Jacob.

Think about taking your first morning breath. It happens every day, and we don't even realize it. We open our eyes, aware and awake, and we breathe. It's such a simple, instinctive act, one that we take for granted, but one that's not easy for Jacob. As his disease progresses, his breathing becomes more labored and he has difficulty managing his secretions. After a long night lying down, movements of awakening seem to stir the fluids around in his chest. As a result, in the mornings, suctioning is often necessary to help clear the pooling secretions in his throat. As he struggles for air, there is terror in his eyes.

And then it happens. He takes in and lets out a long, deep, satisfied breath. Soon to follow, a massive smile breaks across his face as if to say, "Here I am! I made it! Bring on the new day!"

Every new day is a celebration for Jacob. For 19 years, I have had the opportunity to sit in the passenger seat and watch my child as he celebrates the little things in life, and there are so many. That first full breath of air in the morning. The morning forehead kiss from his mother, father or caregiver. The sweet voices of his sister and brother greeting him. A song playing on the radio. As I watch, I learn. Jacob reminds me to focus on the details rather than allowing them to just slide by in a blur. This is a boy who actually does what the cliché insists is the right way to live: He stops and smells the roses. And he does so automatically, without effort. It's a gift he was born with, and one that I try to emulate.

How? Whenever I can, I celebrate.

Every hug I give is a celebration. Consciously, I hug that much tighter and celebrate the love that is passing between us. When I sip a latte, I bask in the sweet warmth of my favorite nurturing drink as it fills my insides. If there is a goal in sight, I give myself an invisible high-five for reaching it.

Like most of us, I sometimes find myself too focused on doing better, achieving more, and in the process, I forget just how far I have come. Now, I make myself stay aware of what's happening in the present and try to celebrate every step along the way. I can assure you that there will be enough setbacks thrown at us. The least we can do is enjoy life as it unfolds. Doing so makes the journey that much more rewarding. Then, when we reach those massive milestones, we can go ahead and celebrate big time. That's what happened at Jacob's Bar Mitzvah.

The guests were seated—all 250 of them. Jacob had made it to 13 and we were gathered to toast a life, an extraordinary life. Jeff and I were so proud. Our firstborn son had made an important transition in the Jewish tradition—symbolically and physically—from childhood to adulthood.

At first, we didn't want to celebrate Jacob's Bar Mitzvah on such a grand scale. We talked about our concerns with our Rabbi, explaining that we wanted to honor Jacob's life but in a small, intimate way.

Our Rabbi nodded and said he understood. He had a question, though. "Why deprive so many people—so many people who love Jake—of the chance to celebrate such a monumental date with him?"

Jeff and I sat in silence as we digested the Rabbi's words. This milestone was not just a celebration of a life. It was the celebration of Jake's life—a celebration of life itself.

Now, the day had arrived. The guests were chatting among themselves, having finished the celebratory lunch. Once the last of the dishes was cleared, Jeff and I hoisted Jacob in his reclined wheelchair onto the stage. We then took our seats on either side of him and we each raised one arm and wrapped it behind our son's shoulders in an embrace. Jacob grinned.

Taking turns speaking, Jeff and I pointed out the tea light and matchbook at each guest's place setting. On the matchbook cover was a small imprint of Jacob's open hand, buttery soft but awkwardly distorted by his unforgiving illness. Below the image were these words: Thank you for being a light in my life. Next to each matchbook sat a tea light just waiting for its wick to shine.

Jeff began. "We look around this room today and we are so blessed to have all of you in Jacob's life. We would love to celebrate today's miracle with a candle-lighting ceremony, but we couldn't choose just 13 people to do the honors because you are all such a support and comfort to us. Many of you will cross over different aspects of Jacob's life, but when you hear the one story that fits you best, please light the small candle in front of you. This is a symbolic way for Jacob to show you how grateful he is that you light up his world."

We took turns telling stories. Some of the stories were serious, some were funny; all were heartwarming, and with each one told, candles were lit and guests were smiling and nodding. One after another, throughout the room, blazing light appeared, just as the stars come out at night. Very soon, the room was ablaze. Jacob beamed—the brightest star of all.

Next, it was 11-year-old Beverly's turn. Jake's sister walked onstage, guitar in hand, and settled herself on a stool. She leaned into the microphone. She and a family friend had composed a song to commemorate this occasion and to honor her big brother. Bev's face was golden and strong in the candlelight. She shot Jacob a quick grin. Then she addressed the audience.

"This is for my brother Jake," she explained and started to sing.
    When I'm feeling blue, just one look at you.
    Smiling in your chair, without a worry or a care.
    You make me realize, my problems are so small in size,
    Jake where would we be without you.
    Oh Jake, I just love you so much.

Within seconds, I was a blubbering mess, my vision drowning in tears of joy and pride, and then I realized, it was contagious. It felt like the room was sobbing.

Behind us, at the back of the stage, was an enormous screen. Jacob's uncle had prepared a surprise. Suddenly, we heard the opening bars of The Beatles' classic *A Little Help from My Friends*. A burst of laughter erupted as the words crossed the screen: *An I Love Jake Film* presents…

What came next was a video montage of Jake's life, starting with photos of him as a baby and morphing one by one into the boy-man he had already become. I watched the show as an outsider looking in as it unspooled, larger than life itself, on the screen before us. I wasn't sad. I was so proud of this young man who thrives against all odds. Proud that he could live a life of fulfillment and manage to give so many such joy. Proud of the dignity and love that somehow surrounds him every second of every day.

The best part is that it's not just his family members who are the beneficiaries of that love. I can't help but notice that everyone around Jake is always smiling. Always. Jeff and I. Jake's younger brother Ben and his sister Bev. His grandparents, cousins, friends, doctors, nurses, teachers and counsellors, and everyone who comes in contact with him.

By all accounts, our child is supposed to be living a tragic life, but everyone in his orbit is always smiling. Somehow, someway, we are doing something right.

Jake's cousins and siblings took turns on the film, narrating on Jacob's behalf. If he were able to speak, these are the words that he might say:

> Thank you for coming to my Bar Mitzvah. In this room, on this special day, are the people who provided me with the non-traditional gift of life. One that has been well documented. Today, there will be no background-style documentary music, nor will I replay the story of my life. You have all seen it, and we have all lived it. Instead, I would like to document the people around me and tell each and every one of you how lucky I am to have you in my life.

Then there was a sudden change in tone. "By the way, please make sure you have a cocktail and are comfortable because the stage is mine and I have been waiting a long time for this opportunity."

Emotions ran deep and complex as we were led through memories of challenges and triumphs, all highlighting Jake's miraculous life. I remember thinking, Jacob may not have the ability to speak, but his message is being delivered, loud and clear.

As I watched images of our son pass on the screen from a giggling baby to a young man, I could not account for what I felt.

It was something way beyond and far stronger than love. This child of mine has been a force in my life—an immensely powerful force that I cherish and learn from and sometimes can't quite comprehend.

Not one bite was taken from the delectable sweet table that day. No one could eat. No one could speak. Everyone left with stomachs half-filled but hearts stuffed.

And there it is: The key to every formal celebration. Celebrating is not about the flowers, although flowers are beautiful. It's not about the food, although good food is delicious. It's not about the clothes, the hair or the makeup, although it is fun to dress up and feel attractive. The fact is, people may compliment what you wear or enjoy what they eat, but chances are those details won't make a lasting impression. What they will remember is how they felt.

It's so easy to get carried away with all of the details in planning a major celebration because there are so many and each one seems important. But here is where we need to step back and take the macro view. If every event is planned around the love, joy and gratitude you feel, it will always feel like a joyous celebration.

On our son's Bar Mitzvah, the congratulatory message was not the typical one. It was not the usual: We are thankful that today, you are a man. It was, instead: We are blessed that today, you are alive.

Now, as Jacob climbs to his twentieth birthday, I write these words in utter awe and humility that I get to be his mother. Celebrations bring people together. They encourage family and friends to bond, connect and reconnect. When we celebrate, even a little, we live.

How do we celebrate life's precious moments with meaning?

- Remember to give yourself an invisible high-five once in a while. You deserve some recognition for a job well done.
- Don't forget to celebrate how far you've come. Looking back will help power you forward.
- Make your hugs last. When you hug just an extra bit tighter and longer it helps you feel the power of connection.
- When planning a celebration, concentrate on the meaning behind it and focus on the love, joy and gratitude. The details are just details.
- Let your heart plan the party. Your brain will follow. Allow everyone in on how you feel so they can feel the love, too.

LESSON 2

Enjoy the Ride

The secret of life is enjoying the passage of time
Any fool can do it
There ain't nothing to it
Nobody knows how we got to
The top of the hill
But since we're on our way down
We might as well enjoy the ride
— James Taylor, *The Secret O' Life*

One day, Jacob and I, and his 10-year-old brother, Ben, were taking a drive on a country road. Jacob was in the back. Our van had been rigged with a ramp to accommodate his wheelchair as well as cleats that securely locked it in place.

That afternoon, we were off for a mother/sons date to lunch and a movie. Cruising down the highway into the sun, Ben and I were nodding our heads in beat to the music on the radio when suddenly, there was a loud bang from behind. We both turned and saw the same sight at the same time: Jake's wheelchair had somehow flipped completely upside down.

Usually, when I'd glance in the rearview mirror, I'd see Jake's face right there in the middle of two captain chairs. Now, there was no sign of him. All we could see were two wheels facing up in the rear of the van.

I gasped. I had never felt such overwhelming fear. Seeing my shock, Ben froze, too, and without thinking, I spun into action. I didn't even take a second to change lanes or pull over. I couldn't do anything except get to Jake as quickly as humanly possible. I slammed on the brakes, stopped the car, looked at Ben and said, "Please don't move." Still frozen in his seat, he couldn't move, even if he tried.

I leapt out and ran behind the van. Cars were lined up behind us now and a bus driver had pulled over to help. I was frantic; I could hardly breathe. Hysterical, I flung open the hatchback door. Jacob's feet were in the air and his head was on the floor of the van, his body still strapped into his chair.

"Jake!" I shouted. "Jake!"

I think I heard the bus driver ask if everyone was okay. My mind was spinning. Panic was caught in my throat, rising in my chest. I had no words.

That's when I looked directly into Jake's face and I will never forget what I saw. Even upside down, it was very clear: Jake was smiling. It was a bright, delighted smile, the kind of childish grin that says, "Now that was a lot of fun. Can we do it again?" There was no doubt about it. This boy loved his ride.

It took me a second to realize that Jacob must have enjoyed the sensation of falling and flipping over. To most of us, it would have been a nightmare of a ride, but to him, it was a thrill.

What I learned that day is that in some ways, life in a wheelchair is a metaphor for the ride we are all taking through life and, somehow, Jacob has figured out how to enjoy it. Whether it's lying on a lounge chair with the wind's gentle massage on his face and the sun melting warmth into his skin or strolling through a mall absorbing all the hustle and bustle, this boy instinctively enjoys his ride. Along the way, he notices the small pleasures first and those seem to give him the greatest satisfaction.

Often, when I'm feeling stressed out, and my body reacts with a quick heart beat or too much sweat, I will lay down beside Jacob. In just moments, his calmness overpowers my hyperactive energy. My breathing begins to slow and, soon, I feel it begin to match his rhythm. My muscles relax as I retreat into his world, into his tranquility.

As I slow down and breathe, I allow peace to engulf me. All of the little stresses that together feel insurmountable start to ebb and then fade away. A clear picture forms in front of me as I adjust myself to Jacob's lens, which seems to be always in focus.

Of course, it's not always easy to find a way to calm ourselves when we are on the brink of feeling overwhelmed. And yet, there are calming forces all around us. What we need to do is learn to notice opportunities and grab hold of them, especially in times of confusion, frustration or stress. But how?

There are some simple tactics that I use to bring back that
peaceful feeling.

- Do you have a pet? Lay down with your animal, who
  holds no emotional stress in its body, and start stroking.
  In just a few minutes, you'll find that calm energy
  transfer to you.
- Pull the car to the side of the road and listen to that song
  that always seems to launch you back to easier days. Let
  the melody move you and help clear the fog.
- Take a few moments to breathe in through your nose and
  out through your mouth. Take in good air, breathe out
  bad. Feel everything around you and inside you slowing
  down.
- Go hug someone you love. Ask if you can make it a long,
  tight hug and then when you're inside it, count to 20.
  Feel the love, accept the comfort, let a few giggles come
  on to ease your pain.

LESSON 3

When We Give, We Live

Try to be a rainbow in someone's cloud.

– Maya Angelou

It may sound trite but it's true: Giving is the best gift of all. In this "I want, I want" world, where everything seems to start with the letter "i"— the iPads, the iPhones—the "you" has to be in there somewhere. Yes, we all love the selfie. But how about we turn that camera around for a change, away from the almighty I? Let's look at what's going on around us, make a contribution—and see what comes back.

Today's companies are taking on social responsibility commitments and our schools are focused on teaching children about community involvement. Why? Simply put, giving feels good. Giving makes us feel like better people. Giving is contagious and meaningful. Random acts of kindness and generosity of the soul will guide us through any of life's uncertainties and challenges. In his book *The Power of Kindness: The Unexpected Benefits of Leading a Compassionate Life*, Piero Ferrucci writes, "Kind people are healthier and live longer, are more popular and productive, have greater success in business and are happier than others." Imagine that.

Often we frown upon the takers in this world, but the fact is, without taking, how can we give? We need givers and accepters for the cycle to continue.

There are so many times when I could have taken help or reached out for help, but I refused. I wanted to be strong, resilient and independent. I was addicted to being the strong one, the woman who can do it all. I see now that I have great difficulty taking. But giving? Now, that's easy.

And guess what I realized? Giving actually makes me a taker as well. Because when I give, I receive something powerful back.

Jacob is a natural receiver. He has no choice; he is helplessly dependent on his caregivers for all necessities in life. He graciously accepts hugs, smiles, kind voices and warm touches. In return, we who give to Jake receive as well. We feel his appreciation and gratitude. We give to him and every time his reaction of joy gives us back more than we could ever give. Here's a prime example.

Many a Sunday at 5 pm, the doorbell rings at the Schwartz house. There stand Stacy and Jennifer, twin sisters with twin smiles on their faces and guitars in hand. Both are leaders in their respective fields of business and mothers to their own children. But here they are at our house, before dinner, every Sunday. It's concert time for Jake.

In the sisters march to the family room where Jacob sits in his reclining wheelchair waiting for his weekly serenade. Stacy picks up her guitar and strums three familiar chords. In response, Jacob's lips curve into a smile. With each note, his smile widens and his eyes sparkle. No words are necessary; the connection and magic of the musical notes do the talking.

For an hour, Stacy, Jennifer and Jake make music. In perfect harmony, the giving cycle is in effect.

Stacy and Jennifer give, Jake graciously receives and gives back. When listening to music, most people sway, tap their feet, nod their heads or sing along. Jacob's eyes brighten as his soul feels the music, but it is the same cycle of giving. As the sisters leave, there is an interesting twist, one that illustrates the giving cycle. They always hug Jacob and thank *him* for making *their* week.

On our emotional road to acceptance, I learned to give. When I gave, I felt better, clearer, more empowered. Perhaps it happened because by giving, I was diverting the focus from my own life and throwing it upon the happiness of others. But giving doesn't come easily to everyone. What if we don't know how to give to someone in need?

Believe it or not, sometimes words are not necessary. Keep in mind that when we can't seem to find the words, a smile and hug will do the talking for us. In fact, sometimes we get lost in words. In trying to read between the lines, we confuse their intended meaning and misinterpret. How many times have you mistaken someone's intention in an e-mail or text? In today's online world, it's so easy to misunderstand, even with emoticons on hand to help.

So what is the right way to react when someone needs help? What are the right words to say? How can we give so the other person will want to receive?

I have learned that sometimes words are not enough. Action is everything. If the right words don't come, try active listening or a connection through eye contact and a supportive smile. These gestures help the other person by communicating good intention. Good intentions are always appreciated, even if we say the wrong thing or our timing is off. If you feel it, chances are, others will too.

But being well meaning is not enough. Often, people ask this question: What can I do to help? This question is not as helpful as it seems. As a person who thinks she can do it all (I really can't), I rarely take anyone up on this "offer" and I'm pretty sure that most people in need also can't answer it.

Why? Think about it. When I am overwhelmed and all wrapped up in life challenges, it's almost impossible to think of ways that other people can help ease the burden. I am trying to survive moment to moment, specifically not focusing on the future. The last thing I want to do in overwhelming moments is to share my burden or unload my pain. The question, while well meaning, comes off more as an obligatory comment than a real offer. And let's face it, if I told you what I really need, you might sprint in the other direction.

What is the right thing to do? Rather than passing the buck with the question, ask yourself this one: What would you need in a similar situation? Get creative now. If you were in that person's shoes, what type of supportive act would you appreciate from a friend? Is it a homemade meal? Is it a carpool drive? Is it walking the dog? Is it grocery shopping? Is it just an ear? Is it a friend to take you out? Is it tulips? A card? Think about what it might be, and deliver.

Once the person you are helping sees action, rather than your words, that's when validation comes. Having experienced your support, the person in need now realizes that your offer to help is legitimate and might even ask for a particular favor in the future.

When Jacob was first diagnosed with Canavan Disease, a friend of mine dropped off a gift in our doorway. It was a binder filled with information about Canavan Disease. She had spent an evening researching Jacob's diagnosis and prognosis. In that moment, and in the hard weeks and months to come, I couldn't think of anything that would have helped more than answers at our doorstep at a time of confusion. Had my friend asked how she could help, I never would have come up with the idea.

Not long ago, a friend of Jacob's passed away. The kids had been in the same class since preschool so they had shared 15 years of life. Jacob had lost his oldest friend and I was struck with grief for her family and for Jacob. I was also suddenly scared for Jacob's future. My gut reaction was to hide in my house and pretend it hadn't happened but there was no way I could retreat. I had to comfort this lovely family at such a tragic time. But I was in need, too.

One of my girlfriends knew instinctively how to give. On the morning of the funeral, she appeared at my door. She drove with me all the way there and sat by my side through the sadness. She knew what I needed even if I didn't.

We had a similar experience with Jeff's brother. Being so close to us, he knew that our nights were daunting and difficult. So one evening, he showed up at our door prepared to stay up all night caring for Jacob, so we could get some rest. And just the other day, I came home to a dozen tulips all wrapped up and propped against my front door. The note read, "Just Because." This kind gesture made my heart sing.

Through these beautiful acts of kindness, given freely by others, I have learned an important lesson: Taking is completely necessary, and not just for me. As I take, the giver is empowered.

Amazed by the kind actions of others, I am inspired to keep giving as well. When I want to help, I just do. I don't wait for the answer. Even if my actions are not always necessary, I know that the message is received: I care and I will help. I don't just want to help. I will help.

Give whenever you can and don't be afraid to take, when you need it most. When you do, you are allowing the cycle of giving to circulate. You are empowering everyone.

How do we keep the giving cycle in motion?
- Remember that action is everything. Don't ask, just do!
- Try not to think too much about what you can do to help. Consider what you would want in the same situation, and just do whatever you think that person will need. Chances are, your instincts are right on target.

- Keep in mind that the question "What can I do to help?" is usually unhelpful. More often than not, it will be met with the answer "Nothing."
- If you're overthinking what to do for someone, remind yourself that the only gesture that won't be appreciated is no gesture at all.
- Be prepared to accept help from others. By taking, you are not the only one benefitting from kindness. You are helping them as well.

LESSON 4

Embrace Teachable Moments

When one feels seen and appreciated in their own essences,
one is instantly empowered.

— Wes Angelozzi

I am a teacher through and through. There is no greater feeling than seeing that lightbulb turn on in a child's eyes. The best lessons are the ones that aren't planned, the ones that grow organically from a comment or a question. Those are the moments when you can inspire a room full of students to be better people.

You don't have to be a teacher to experience teachable moments. As parents, we live these moments every day and it's our job to seize them. It's our job to make sure we don't let the opportunity to teach pass us by. What we need to do, every day, is take the time to model life lessons, whenever possible. It is these lessons that children will remember and pass on to others.

As a teacher, I wanted the opportunity to teach lessons that could last a lifetime. It doesn't matter how old we are or where we are from, we each have a story to share, one that can make an impact. I saw what happened when I shared Jacob's story, and I wanted to make it a richer experience for everyone involved by growing the pie, by creating a space where we can all learn from each other.

How? I launched Project Give Back, a year-long curriculum geared for elementary students. The program is designed to help them develop empathy, build character and to inspire them to become community-minded young adults. Because children make a difference in the lives of others by sharing their own life experiences, Project Give Back is based on sharing and giving.

The premise is simple. Together with their family members, each student finds a cause that they are passionate about, and this cause becomes the topic of their year-long Project Give Back journey. Each student reaches out to make that initial connection. They go on to research their charity, write a speech about it and share what they learn with the rest of us.

The first class begins with a brainstorming session where students call out the names of various charities they know. I remember when one student called out the MS Read-a-thon. "What a great cause!" I said. "And who do they help?" The child answered, "People with cancer."

Helping is great, but imagine how much better it would feel if we understood exactly who it is we are helping—and why. Through Project Give Back, children become classroom experts on their chosen topic. Then, they share their expertise with the rest of us—their classmates, teachers and family members. From our students, we learn about the world through their lenses.

Each year, more than 1,000 students now take on more than 500 causes that have touched them personally. We all know if we follow our hearts and passion, people listen but we have to take action to really spread goodness.

As teachers and parents, we know that curiosity begets knowledge. Familiarity brings acceptance. Sharing leads to empathy and compassion. These values all come alive in Project Give Back as children learn from one another, giving and receiving.

Project Give Back's logo is a boomerang with a star inside— and for good reason. I love asking the students what they think the logo means.

Why the boomerang? Because when you throw it out there, it comes back.

What are we throwing out there into the world? Acts of kindness.

Why is there a star inside of the boomerang? Because each one of us has a star inside waiting to shine.

The students are right. As each child gives, shares and spreads their knowledge, everyone shines brighter, and that's what giving is all about.

Looking for the right educators for our team wasn't easy. Each one had to be a worldly, parental, inspirational, motivational role model and of course, a qualified teacher as well. They had to believe in each child's abilities and know they had the means to reach each child. The Project Give Back lessons they taught had to be ones that they themselves had learned through their own unique experiences. Slowly and carefully, our team was built with teachers who love what they do, and the results illustrate their efforts.

Here are a few Project Give Back teachable moments.

Right from her first Project Give Back session, Sloane knew which cause had touched her heart. Without a doubt, she knew what she wanted to share and how she wanted to share it. After initiating a relationship with Mount Sinai Hospital, Sloane never looked back. She worked tirelessly to do her best, and succeeded.

Sloane's mother had spent a very hard year both in and out of Mount Sinai Hospital in Toronto. Her illness had taken its toll on the family and in Sloane's mind, Project Give Back was just the right way to turn a challenging situation into a positive one.

The date of Sloane's presentation arrived. She had reached out to her charity. She had completed her research. She had written her speech and practiced it many times over. Now was her day to shine.

She stood at the front of the classroom ready to inspire. Confidently and with pride, Sloane spoke about her mother's battle with ulcerative colitis and her gratitude for the hospital that helped her family. She showed photographs of birthdays, anniversaries and holidays spent at her mother's hospital bedside. She spoke about the nurses who lovingly cared for her mother.

Silence filled the room as Sloane spoke about her mother's battle. Our hearts reached out to her as she spoke honestly, with knowledge and expertise. Together, all of the students in the class made thank you cards for the nurses at Mount Sinai Hospital.

Sloane's shining moment impacted so many lives—her classmates, the nurses and, of course, her family. Because her lesson came from the heart, it made a real and lasting impact.

Four years later, Sloane is one of the youngest committee members planning the Gutsy Walk, a fund-raising event for Crohn's and Colitis Canada.

When children teach, we sit up and listen and, often, one child will inspire another to share, creating a sort of domino effect.

One boy spoke about Nellie's Place, a shelter providing safety and support to women and children in crisis. It was a tough lesson for anyone to learn, especially kids. One boy listened to the presentation then bravely raised his hand. When called upon, he surprised everyone by sharing the details of his own personal experience living in a shelter.

Everyone listened intently as he spoke about his own crisis and the shelter that helped his family. And as he shared, feeling safe enough to speak about something so personal, his friends rallied around him. They marveled at his courage. "No therapy could help him, but this worked," his mother told me. Hence, the power of giving.

And then there was a boy, we will call Henry. Henry taught a lesson that many of us will never forget. It was his day to be the teacher and he took on his role with gusto. He stood at the front of the room and led the class in a song with actions to fit the words. All of the children were engaged, clapping, moving and flapping their arms to the lyrics.

Afterward, he instructed everyone to sit still and listen. Before he started, he asked one classmate to flick the lights on and off in rapid succession while he spoke. Then Henry began his speech about The Geneva Centre for Autism. It was almost impossible to listen with the lights flickering on and off and on and off.

Finally, the teacher shouted "STOP!"

Henry stopped. The lights stopped. The children sat motionless. Henry said, "This is how my brother feels all of the time. He has autism."

Henry went on to speak about autism and how it affects his brother. This eight-year-old boy took the complex idea of empathy and made it the basis of his presentation. Through his leadership and direction, we were able to feel, if only for a moment, what it must be like to be autistic. We were all confused, disorientated and frustrated. All of us, moved.

After Henry's lesson, he invited a special guest to come up to join him. It was his younger brother with autism. We all sang the song Henry had taught us at the beginning of the class and his brother cheered with joy that this whole group of children had learned his favorite song. He was smiling and clapping along.

Months later, I received a call from Henry's mother. She had received a call from a woman she had never met. One day, some young girls came over to play with this woman's daughter. She has autism. When the woman finally mustered the nerve to ask these young girls what prompted them to come over, they recounted the details of Henry's presentation. After listening to it, it occurred to them that their neighbor reminded them of Henry's brother. They figured she might like some visitors, and they were right.

Teachable moments happen at unexpected times and at unexpected moments. They are rarely planned, but they are always dramatically impactful.

Another example is brave Sam who spoke about his own battle with Tourette Syndrome. Months after his project was through, Sam decided that he was going to help advocate for the cause. Here is an article that Sam wrote.

> When I first heard of *it* … all I knew about *it* …was that I might have *it*! *Tourette Syndrome* – What the tic was Tourette Syndrome? I thought. My mom told me that she was worried about the fact that I might have Tourette Syndrome. At first, I didn't really take her seriously because she worries all the time.
>
> The first time *it* happened, I was seven years old. I was playing Monopoly with my mom. I randomly had the urge to start saying some made up words. I began to say some of these weird words…That was when *it* all started…I had these verbal tics for a few months and then over the course of the next few years, varying disruptive tics intruded on my life and they still do today.
>
> Around the same time, I was participating in a school play and I asked my mom if I could drop out. My tics were making me uncomfortable and I didn't want people to notice them. My mom encouraged me to

continue, as I had already committed to the play. In the end, I was glad my mom forced me to do it because I enjoyed the experience and my tics were temporarily nonexistent while I was performing.

Except for my closest friends, I didn't tell very many people about the fact that I had Tourette Syndrome, as I found it to be slightly embarrassing. Things stayed like that until fifth grade when my class was assigned a project called Project Give Back. This is a project that many students in grades four and five all around Toronto participate in. We would choose a charity to tell the class about and in each presentation, there would be a little game representing what the charity does.

Having Tourettes, I automatically chose the TFSC as the charity for my project. It just felt right. I explained about Tourette Syndrome and how it can affect your life. For another part of the presentation, I told my classmates that I did indeed have Tourettes. The kids didn't react badly at all. They just accepted it as if everything was normal. I didn't feel embarrassed during my presentation, so it was then that I realized that I was starting to feel okay with telling people that I had Tourette Syndrome! No one is going to judge me just because I have this disorder.

Everyone was very impressed with my presentation, and my teachers suggested that I show it to other children around the city to raise awareness about Tourette

Syndrome. Raising awareness is important so that people know about Tourettes and how it can affect one's life. It can also show people that I am not weird. I feel completely normal even though I have Tourettes. It was not until quite recently, however, that I actually stepped up and decided that I wanted to be an advocate.

Just recently, Sam published his first book of poetry called *Insights*. The funds raised from sales will go directly to Tourette Canada, a charity dedicated to creating awareness and understanding of Tourette Syndrome.

Life is filled with these teachable moments that enhance our lives. We just have to grasp them, turn a blind eye to our own predetermined judgments and let the learning seep through. When it comes to learning and teaching, we are all students as well as teachers.

How can we make sure we don't let teachable moments pass us by?

- Think of your own teachable moments. There's that moment when you realized why you failed. When you realized there is something to be learned here. That moment when you pushed yourself more than you ever thought possible. That moment when you picked up the pieces and forged ahead.

- Remember that we have a responsibility to each other to be generous with those moments and to share them. That way, they will impact someone else and we will all learn

and grow from each other's lessons. When we share, we
all benefit.

- Open your eyes to the unlimited number of teachable
  lessons that surround you every moment of the day.
  Every time you learn from one, write it down so you can
  let it out into the world.
- Each one of us has many stories to tell. Become an open
  book so we can learn from you and continue to gain
  insight, understanding and knowledge.
- When a teachable moment happens, find a new way to
  pass it on. The domino effect spreads learning and makes
  the world a better place.
- Don't be afraid to share your passion with others. If you
  are truly passionate about something, it usually means
  that you are the expert in the room on that particular
  subject. Be prepared to share your insight so everyone
  can benefit.

LESSON 5

You Don't Have to Speak to be Heard

Too often we underestimate the power of a touch,
a smile, a kind word, a listening ear,
an honest compliment,
or the smallest act of caring,
all of which have the potential to turn a life around.

– Leo Buscaglia

Great teachers come in all shapes, sizes, and ages and the best ones aren't always found in the classroom. That's because the most impactful lessons are not always taught. Instead, they are lived.

If we want students to share, it is imperative that we share with them. I share Jacob. I wheel him into the classroom, unannounced. The students have all heard of Jacob. They have seen photos of him and listened to his story, but something changes when they meet him face to face. Let's just say, he can silence a kid-filled room in a fraction of a second, which is not an easy task when those kids are only ten years old.

At first glance, the students are startled and exhibit a range of mixed emotions. Some are clearly put off. Some look scared. Many are wide-eyed, full of open curiosity. One thing is clear: This experience is new. Rarely has anyone met a child with such severe disabilities.

Jacob and I take our position at the head of the class. His wheelchair is large and daunting, so I bend my knees and carefully slip one arm behind his neck and squeeze the other beneath his knees. As the kids watch, I pull Jacob close and lift him onto my lap. His legs rest on my legs, and my arm is strategically placed between his head and neck in order to support him. I ask the children to come and join us. Some run up, clearly eager to meet Jacob while others take their time, hoping for a seat at the rear. We are now at their level. The children watch in silent fascination as I introduce my son.

"Class, we have a very special visitor today. Please meet Jacob."

Quiet, reluctant whispers: "Hi Jacob."

I ask the students a simple question. "I am just wondering if anyone feels a little uncomfortable right now but cannot pinpoint why you feel that way? If you do, just take your finger and press it against your chest."

All fingers immediately tap away at their own chests.

I nod and smile. "Me too!" I say. I can tell some of the kids don't believe me.

"It's true." My aim is to validate the children's feelings because emotions are important pieces of information. I want them to understand that it's okay to feel discomfort. I know because I used to feel the same. I ask them why they think they feel this way. Half-raised hands slowly lift.

"Because we have never met anyone like this before."

"Because he's so different from us."

"I'm not sure why, but I feel funny."

I can feel the atmosphere thaw as the kids warm to having Jacob in their presence. The emotional walls are already sliding down. I tell them about my life before Jacob was born and explain that the way they are feeling—the way they were feeling at first—is exactly how I felt. I hadn't met anyone like Jacob before, either. I didn't know how to speak to someone who wasn't able to speak back.

As Jacob feels my cuddles and listens to the sweet voices from the students, his eyes widen and his smile appears. I ask the students, "Do you think Jacob is happy or sad?"

"So happy. He likes it here," one student replies.

"How can you tell he's so happy?" I probe. "He didn't tell you that."

Another student raises his hand and says, "You can see it in his eyes. And look at his smile. His smile says it all."

Slowly, the students begin to lean in to learn more. Pretty soon, their hands are shooting up. The tone has turned from reluctance to confidence—even acceptance. I let them know that it's okay to fire off any questions they have about Jacob. Anything at all. The only question that is wrong is the one that isn't asked. With all barriers removed, hands start flying in the air.

"Why do his teeth look so funny?" asks one student.

I answer honestly. "When you can't use muscles, they grow in funny looking. Jake isn't able to eat with his teeth, so they grow in differently than yours."

"How does he eat?"

I uncover his feeding machine and explain that it contains everything nutritious that Jacob's body needs. I show them the bag that holds his liquid food and how it is placed into the feeding pump. I show them the long tube attached to the pump and tell them we insert a similar tube into Jacob's stomach. I explain that the food bypasses his mouth and goes directly to his stomach. This last statement is usually followed by ooohs and ahhhs. Kids this age think this is just about the coolest process they have ever witnessed. Then I let them know that Jacob can even eat when he sleeps. Now jaws are downright open. No one can believe that Jacob has such talents.

"Does anyone want to try Jacob's food to see what it tastes like?"

One student reluctantly volunteers. He puts out his hand and another student pushes the start button on the feeding pump. With that, a small white drop of liquid falls into his palm. We push the stop button to end the feed. The student raises his palm to his mouth and hesitantly licks the drop.

"Yum! It tastes so good, just like a vanilla milkshake."

By this time, the students have jumped up from the floor and have moved closer to Jacob. Jacob is grinning because he knows he has just made many new friends. There is no more raising of hands, just a rapid fire of random questions.

What does Jacob do for fun? What is his favorite activity? Does he sleep in his chair? Does he have friends? Will he get married? Is he heavy? What's his middle name? Does he go to school? What school? What's his best friend's name?

One by one, all questions are answered.

They want to know what types of music Jacob likes to listen to. I explain that like everyone, he does have particular musical taste. For instance, he loves Bruno Mars and Adele. The next thing we know, Jacob is being serenaded by a classroom of students singing *The Lazy Song*. A smile spreads across Jacob's face and the children giggle with pride. Although Jacob hasn't said a word, they see that they have contributed to his happiness.

By this time, I'm tired from holding up Jacob with only my arm and legs. I stand and carefully place him back in his chair. The students surround him and ask if they can take him for a walk. I ask them to sit back down with us first. As they lean in to listen, I ask why they think I brought Jacob in to meet them. What lessons did they learn? The answers always take me by surprise—they are so pure, honest and accepting.

"We learned that we can't judge a book by its cover."

"Just because Jacob looks different, doesn't mean he is different."

"He's just like us and I made a new friend today."

Unfortunately, due to Jacob's progressing illness, we have had to take a break from visiting classes. Fortunately, though, many of our visits were taped so future classes will still get the opportunity to meet Jacob and to be transformed by the experience.

Just by experiencing inclusion that leads to understanding, these children will grow up not fearing people who are different. Their feelings of acceptance, compassion and empathy, which grow from a foundation of understanding, will travel with them through life. As they spread these feelings in the world, they will participate in changing the lives of everyone they meet.

Jacob was able to teach a lesson that no textbook, web page or teacher could ever convey. And it's important to realize that this enrichment happened without Jacob uttering even one word.

There are so many ways that we can enrich our own lives without the need for words but in our busy world, it's easy to miss those valuable opportunities. How can we make sure we get the most out of the signs and signals that the world has to offer? We do it every day; we just don't always realize it.

How do we read the signs when there aren't any words? How can we understand someone else, when they don't let us know how they are feeling?

Every day, we obey signs. We stay a certain distance from the driver in front of us because we know that's safe. We stop at red lights and move forward on green.

A look, a voice, a touch—these are all important communication tools. Just one glance into our children's eyes and we know what's up. Somehow, we know what to do to make them feel better. I rarely call my own parents when I feel deflated because I know that just from the tone of my voice, they will know. But what about everyone else in our life? We aren't mind readers—or are we?

Often my children make fun of me because I take so long to say goodbye when it's time to leave. I am connecting, trying to feel people from the inside.

Have you ever bumped into an acquaintance and found that their words do not match their smile? When I do, we engage in the usual polite chit-chat and then it's obvious. I can feel there is something else behind the words. It's in the tone of their voice and their body language. They say one thing, but they are conveying something else.

"So how are you?" I ask.

"I'm great," comes the answer, but instinctively I know different.

There is a nod of understanding between us, without one word spoken. Sometimes the result is a glaze over the eyes with barely perceptible tears that show real emotions bubbling over. That little gesture is a thank you. To know that someone gets you is a very motivating feeling. It can change a life, or at least put a skip into their day.

How do we connect with people around us, even if they don't express themselves through words?

- Whether you are at the grocery store, the bank, the gym or the subway, look up and around. Catch the eyes of the people who surround you. Doing so allows you to live in the moment and make connections with others.

- Look into the eyes of strangers, acquaintances and friends, and be open to what you see and more importantly how you feel.
- Remember that touch is a powerful connector. A touch on the arm or a shoulder-to-shoulder rub conveys the message that you identify with someone else.
- Take your time saying hello and goodbye.
- Read body language because it tells a lot about how people feel. If you think you may have missed a friendly cue from someone's body language, send an e-mail or text letting the person know that you are thinking about them. This small gesture confirms that you care.

LESSON 6

Open Up to Unexpected Friendships

You can count on me like 1, 2, 3 – I'll be there.
I can count on you like 4, 3, 2, you'll be there.
Cuz that's what friends are supposed to do, oh yeah.

— Bruno Mars

Ten years ago, over dinner with a close girlfriend, I opened up and blurted out some truths. I told her that while I loved teaching Project Give Back, I felt like I was burning out. I was head of administration (not my strong suit), tweaking the curriculum, teaching 16 classes a week, writing more than 30 reports and trying to run my household in what was starting to feel like very little spare time. Something had to give before I collapsed.

My girlfriend looked at me and then gave me one of the greatest gifts I have ever received, the gift of her time. She would run the office and administration so I wouldn't have to. A graduate from the University of Pennsylvania and an MBA grad from Northwestern University, this friend was beyond qualified to grow the business side of our charity. The problem was, I didn't have the money to pay her. But that didn't seem to matter.

Fast forward to today. This same friend continues to donate her time, energy and resources to helping to run Project Give Back. She does so with boundless energy, smarts and a smile, and all out of the kindness of her heart—free of charge.

We can never underestimate the value of friendship. True friends are priceless. They build us up, rejoice in our joy and empower us in our most vulnerable moments. Just like teachable moments, the best of friends can be unexpected. They can enter your life at any time. You just have to be wise enough to recognize them.

The fact is, you never know who might have an impact on your life or the extent to which a person can change you. Jacob's friendships are deep and meaningful. They aren't based on first impressions. They are true connections of the soul. Jacob is picky; he draws in certain people who connect with him for a specific time frame, but because the friendships are real, they remain bonded forever.

Emily is one of those friends. When Jacob and Emily met, she was a music specialist at Bayview Glen Day Camp. Jacob's face lit up every time he heard this girl strumming away on her guitar. So much so that Jake's two camp counselors wheeled him around to follow Emily. He was her number-one fan. Although they couldn't converse in words, they shared a similar language: Music.

Emily wrote about her connection with Jacob in her thesis, "The Limitless Powers of Music: A Disabled Child Finds Peace in Sound."

Here is an excerpt:

Jacob is twelve now. He still cannot speak, see, eat, or support himself, but he can hear. He attends a school that meets his needs. He certainly knows how to enjoy the simple things in life, and he can teach. He is a constant reminder to people around him of how to enjoy the simplest things in life and never take anything for granted. It's absolutely amazing to experience spending time with someone who can teach you so much without ever saying a word.

Since hearing is the one main sense that Jacob hasn't lost, music has always been particularly powerful with him. According to Ellen, music saved Jacob's life when he was two years old and in a coma. Just when his parents were about to give up hope, the instructor of a music class Jacob used to attend sent them a CD. Her little gift prompted Ellen to call and ask her to come and play to Jacob in the hospital. As soon as she began to play to him, a smile began to appear on his face. "We knew that Jacob was on his way back to us...All because of the power of music."

Having had the opportunity to meet and play to Jacob myself, I can certainly believe the power music has with him. He expresses himself more than in any other situation I have seen when he hears music he likes: He begins to move, and he even tries to sing along. His favourite kinds of music? Jacob loves all music and all types of music from classical to rock and roll. He truly loves a live performance of acoustic guitar and soft singing.

As it turns out, Jacob is a magnet for the ladies. When he was just seven years old, we received a call from an eleven-year-old girl named Ali. She was new to us all. The conversation went something like this.

"Hello, Ellen?"

"Yes."

"My name is Ali and I would like to spend time with Jacob in preparation for a Bat Mitzvah project that I am working on. Can I come over to spend some time with Jacob and help you out on Sundays?"

That Sunday, we opened our doors to meet sweet Ali. She was so young and yet mature beyond her years. She was excited to meet her new playmate.

Ali and Jacob bonded right away. They giggled together as Ali read to him. They hung out watching TV, holding hands. They went for long walks together, with Ali pushing Jacob's chair. The friendship started with one-hour visits but soon, each visit stretched longer and longer. Eventually, Sundays became Ali days. That meant that she joined us on our family outings. We couldn't help but adopt Ali as our weekend daughter.

Originally, the plan was that these Sunday sessions were supposed to last for eight weeks, but instead, they went on for years. Today, Ali is away at university, but whenever she has a chance, she comes to visit her buddy. Not only did we adopt Ali, but we adopted her family as well.

Ali wrote about her unique friendship with Jacob:

It all started with a Bat Mitzvah project...

Jacob and I met when I was twelve years old. I chose to spend time with Jacob and his family and write about my experiences as a community service and growth opportunity. Every Sunday for eight weeks, I went over to the Schwartz house and got to know Jacob, little by little.

As you can imagine, I was a little timid at first because I had never met anybody like Jacob before. I was unsure how to act around him. Watching his family interact with him and seeing how he responded helped me learn all about the things he enjoyed. When I saw Jacob's *huge* smile, I became more comfortable, and our timid visits soon turned into a great friendship. We would read together, listen to music, go for walks, or do special activities for hours on end. I remember how amazing it felt the first time Jacob recognized my voice and smiled his huge smile as I walked in to greet him.

I knew that I enjoyed spending this time with Jacob and his family, but what I never imagined was that I would continue my Sunday visits to the Schwartz household for the next six years. Hanging with Jacob became part of my weekly routine, and I always looked forward to going to his house on the weekend.

I learned so much about Jacob over the years, from his favourite songs to his feeding and medicine routines. But more importantly, I learned so much from him. Jacob taught me to appreciate the little things in my life, like the sounds and sights around me and all of my own abilities. He taught me the importance of a smile and how easy it is to just be happy and content.

Jacob was a constant reminder to me to minimize my so-called problems and focus on all the positive things in my life. Being around Jacob genuinely made me happy and I believe he has made me a better person. From a young age, I became comfortable around people who were different from myself, and looked past outward appearances. I became passionate about volunteering and helping others.

My friendship with Jacob has been a continuous influence on many of my life's choices. For one, he inspired me to continue learning about and working with individuals with special needs—both children and adults—throughout high school, my gap year in Israel, and into university. As well, I am currently completing a Health Sciences degree at university because someday, I want to help other people like Jakey.

What started as a small project turned into a friendship that has played a lasting role in my life, and I am so thankful to have Jacob in my life.

And then there's Melda, a woman we call Jake's Angel. We met her when she showed up for her first shift as a personal support worker to help around the house. We are always so grateful for the caregivers who visit us on a daily basis. Some take the time to understand Jake's needs while others come to help on their own agendas.

Melda is radiant. Right from hello, you can feel the goodness which fuels her insides. The first time I opened the door to receive Melda, her sincere smile touched mine. We introduced her to Jake. She strode right up to him, put her hand on his heart and said, "Hi Jacob, I am here to be your friend and keep you comfortable and safe."

That was 14 years ago. Since that day, Melda has become our family. Not only is she Jacob's best friend, but she is also my lifeline. I trust her with my child, and with my heart and soul, because I know that she loves him as her own. When Melda is near, he is safe, and my breathing slows down. Like with any true friend, when she is near, I can relax.

Unexpected friendships come at any age.

I'll never forget the day I met Sam. Our family was lunching in a restaurant, Jacob by my side, when I felt a soft kiss on the top of my head. I looked up and there standing over me was an elderly gentleman I had never met. I looked up at him in surprise.

His kind eyes resting on my face, he introduced himself.

"My name is Sam. I have been watching you with your son all through lunch. I couldn't help but notice the way you hold his hand, stroke his leg and constantly kiss his cheek. I needed to meet you so I could let you know how much the love you have for each other has touched me."

Sam's words not only sparked an intimate conversation between two strangers but it also opened up a beautiful friendship to both of us.

Months later, I was speaking at an event about the importance of inclusion, and there, right in the front row, was Sam. He had heard that I was the guest speaker and wanted to be there.

Another surprise visit started with a knock on our door. Sam was standing there on our front stoop holding a special gift he had made for his buddy Jacob. It was a silver ladder with five rungs. On three of the rungs, there were symbols representing Faith, Hope and Charity, referring to Jacob's Ladder connecting Earth to Heaven. Ever since, this ladder has been standing guard by Jacob's bedside.

Like Sam, Uncle Norman was another unexpected friend who graced us with his love and generosity. At the young age of 90, Uncle Norman would visit Jacob's school during the annual holiday concert. He would come bearing gifts, which he would hand deliver to each student. He also brought party-size birthday cakes to the teachers, people that Uncle Norman referred to as angels.

Every year, we could count on Uncle Norman showing up to shower us with his holiday giving until he passed away at the age of 96. Each year, we remember the example of kindness and empathy that he set. It's one that we all hope to emulate.

We never know when or where we will find the deepest of friendships. I am in awe of some of the bonds that didn't form until I hit my 40s. When I think about the new and old friends I am so lucky to be surrounded by, I can't help but tear up. My gratefulness for how precious they are is all-encompassing.

Ever heard this statement? "I really found out who my true friends are, that's for sure." It's usually uttered by someone who has gone through turmoil or tragedy, as I have. The fact is, life's challenges do weed out your friendships. They test the current bonds and create opportunities for more to form.

While many friends and family members have been there for us, others surprised me by failing to offer support. For my part, I make a conscious choice to focus on the people in my life who do step up. Why be disappointed in some friends when you can choose to feel grateful for others instead? Of course, there are times when I can't help but feel let down. Instead of dwelling on those negative thoughts, though, I choose to make them temporary, turning my mind to those who make me feel blessed.

I have learned that when we expect something of others, we are setting ourselves up for disappointment. We are counting on a certain reaction, and when it doesn't come, we are let down. Conversely, when we don't expect anything, we are genuinely surprised by the outcome. This lesson is the key to all relationships, and I learned it from my son. Watching Jacob with the people who interact with him, I see that joy comes when you least expect it.

Being open to unexpected friendships will allow them to enter and enrich your life. Here are some ways to let them into your world and keep them there.

- Open your heart to new friendships, no matter what age or stage of your life. If there is a connection, don't doubt it. It's there for a reason.

- Always remember to show your appreciation by kind words or gestures. Successful friendships are based on give and take.
- Never take friendships for granted. Like any living thing, they take work and care.
- Don't go too long without checking in with your friends, whether by phone, e-mail, text or, best of all, in person.
- Don't underestimate the power of gestures. Drop off some homemade soup, cookies or flowers when you feel a friend could use some love.
- Be ready to be a listener rather than jumping to dispensing advice. Very often, a supportive ear is what your friend needs most.

Embrace Our Differences

If you change the way you look at things,
the things you look at change.

– Wayne Dyer

Inclusion. It's a big ol' buzzword these days, and for good reason. Everyone wants to feel included. Everyone needs to feel included. But what does the word mean exactly?

We use the term inclusion to refer to people who are different, often those with special needs. By including them in our framework, we are attempting to normalize experiences for them. What we miss in the process, though, is what we can learn by including people who are different in our life experiences. How can their differences enrich our lives? True inclusion is about people with special needs teaching the world about what life is all about.

"He will never walk."

"He will never talk."

"He will never see."

"He will lose his ability to eat."

"He will lose his ability to breathe."

"He will die before his fifth birthday."

I heard these words 19 years ago. They described Jacob's prognosis. And after they were spoken, I had one burning question I couldn't help but ask. I don't know why. Maybe it was because my childhood summers were storybook in so many ways that I cherish and I wanted my child to feel that sense of inclusion. "But will he go to camp?"

When Jacob was eight years old, a friend and I were chatting about his plans for the summer. Dara directs a day camp for more than a thousand campers, run by more than 400 teenage staff. When the topic came up, she shrugged and informed me that Jacob would, of course, attend Bayview Glen Day Camp. I was stunned. How could Jacob possibly go to a camp that caters to healthy children?

That's when Dara's love and respect of the underdog spoke to me. She had it all figured out. She assured me that nurses would attend to Jacob and two trained counselors would assist with his every need. I would be just a phone call away, she reminded me, and could be reached at any second.

Camp proved to be a life changer for all of us. On his mobile throne, Jacob became a friend to campers of all ages. With his specialized counselors in tow, he could participate in regular activities. He swam, lay on the trampoline and bounced, followed the off-road trails in his wheelchair, enjoyed music classes and finger painted. He even went rock climbing, Jake-style. Hoisted aloft in a specially adapted harness that freed him from his chair,

Jake experienced for the first time the exquisite sensation of floating in the air. The summer transformed everyone.

It wasn't until after camp ended that we stumbled on a special post-camp gift. We were cleaning out Jacob's backpack, which was still sitting in the back of his wheelchair, and we pulled out a letter written by Sapir, a 17-year-old camp counselor.

Dear Jacob,

I don't believe in miracles, yet there is no one who can convince me that you aren't a miracle straight out of heaven. Yes, your smile is contagious and yes, you appreciate life to its fullest and yes, you are the most amazing person I have and will ever meet. But there is something about you that I haven't seen in anybody in my entire life. The way you love people. It's not the fact that you love. It's how you love.

You have so much power to change people. Change their day, change their mood and change their life. I won't ever meet someone who, constantly and no matter what, will simply love.

Thank you for teaching me about the importance and power of love. Thank you for smiling for me when I needed it. Thank you for understanding me and thank you for being there for me. Every moment I spent with you will be cherished by me forever, but there is one scene that is replayed in my head over and over again.

When Emily played guitar and sang Hallelujah for you, the way you reacted is engraved in my heart forever. It wasn't your smile because your smile has been bigger. It wasn't your eyes glowing because they have been wider. It was the look of peace on your face. You were telling stories with your face and not one word came out of your mouth. You were saying, "This is where I need to be, this is what I need."

You don't need the fancy stuff, Jakey. You don't need to swim every day or go rock climbing or play on the drum and pet animals. You just need to connect.

There is no person in the world that has affected me as you have, Jacob, and I will be forever in your debt because of it. Hold on to that dear smile of yours for as long as you can because that's precisely the thing that keeps us all going. I love you very much, Jakey.

Forever yours,

Sapir

At camp, Jacob is Jacob. He doesn't have the ability to be anyone else or to meet anyone else's expectations. He is himself and everyone at camp is attracted to his infectious love of life. Sure, there are the continual jaws dropping as children spot him the for first time. But as questions are asked with curiosity and innocence, they are answered with direct honesty. And what happens next is what's most magical. The intimidating, reclining, black, metal wheelchair disappears and children begin to see the person who proudly sits there. The differences, which tend to dictate how we treat others, no longer matter. At a camp that caters to healthy children, Jacob is accepted, included and loved, and that can happen anywhere.

We had another gift from Jacob's camp experience. Together, his counselors carefully crafted a scrapbook to highlight special camp memories. It was filled with letters from many staff members who each shared memorable moments with Jacob.

> Dear Jacob,
>
> It seems like such a short time ago that Dan and I met you and for the first time and even now I can say with the utmost confidence that you have changed my life for the better. I have learned to appreciate everything and everyone, to be strong and to be confident in who I am as a person.
>
> Thanks Jacob for reminding me to stay positive and live in the moment more. Thank you for inspiring me to be my best each day and for teaching our campers that unique is beautiful.

We had hoped that summer camp would stimulate and inspire Jacob, and it did. What we didn't anticipate were the reciprocal results. While we hoped that without us to protect him, to educate and explain, he would not be shunned, we couldn't imagine the extent to which he might be embraced.

We are all aware of the way in which we judge others based on appearance. After all, in this new world of selfies posted everywhere, it's hard not to be critical. But as parents of a special needs child, we are even more attuned to the reality of judgment and discrimination based on the fear of differences.

Imagine if these barriers could be broken down everywhere, if society ran just like this amazing summer camp and, in the world at large, if we could embrace one another's differences and uniqueness? It won't happen without education, familiarity and understanding.

Recently, I was wandering around in the mall with my two sons when Ben asked, "Mom, why does everyone stare?"

My answer came in a sarcastic but loving tone, "Well Ben, not all 18-year-olds have that awesome flow of red hair that Jacob has."

We both giggled then created a game. Every time someone shot Jacob an open-mouthed glare, Ben and I shot each other a grin.

Often, I take Jacob grocery shopping with me. I know we are a sight to behold. It's impossible not to notice when people turn on their heels and walk the other way. More than once, a mother will say to her kids, nice and loud, "Be careful honey, don't go too close." Although understandable, the fear is difficult to take. Many people don't know how to react when faced with someone who is different, and the lack of education is to blame.

This excerpt from an article in *The Globe and Mail* newspaper written by the mother of a child with autism gets to the heart of the problem. What she sees as her child's ability to view the world through a loving lens is lost on the people around her. If we could all see with this child's perspective, just think of the world that we could all enjoy.

> I am jealous that a person could be so ecstatic while waiting in line at a Superstore. I wish I knew what makes her so happy so I could be that happy too. I'll just have to be happy watching her. The other shoppers are not happy. The mothers hide their children. Some pretend not to watch. Some watch with disgust. I watch with envy.

That's it right there. What we all need is the ability to celebrate our special population. In that way, we can learn to open our minds to a different world, a better world.

Did you see the viral video of Sam, a 17-year-old Starbucks barista with autism? To date, there have been millions of views of this young man singing and dancing as he brews specialty coffees. Here's a not-so-fun fact: Sam's parents were told that he would never be employable. The experts were proven wrong. Not only did Sam get a job, but he managed to make it all the way to *The Ellen Show*. In her interview with Sam, Ellen DeGeneres asked him what it was like to be hired for a job. Sam answered, "In that moment, my life changed, my whole world changed."

In fact, by hiring Sam, that Starbucks manager did something he probably couldn't anticipate. He changed the lives of all those customers lucky enough to be on the receiving end of this young man's coffee creations. What a way to start off the day, coffee with a dance and a smile! Put me in that line any day.

At the 2016 Grammy Awards, millions watched as Stevie Wonder stood on the stage and said, "We need to make every single thing accessible to every single person with a disability." That's a laudable goal, but I say we need to take it a step further. It is not only people with disabilities who need acceptance. It's all of us. Whether we are talking about a plus-size radiant model on the cover of *Sports Illustrated*, a young beauty with Down Syndrome taking over the fashion runways or a young Jacob at summer camp, everyone is deserving of our respect. No one deserves to be shunned. When we do so, we not only deny them our love, but we miss out on what we can receive in return.

How can we train ourselves to accept people with differences? Here are some ideas you can use to dampen the fear and intimidation you may feel and to allow you to be more inclusive of others.

- A friend once told me that in order to understand others you have to do this: Turn it on its head. While walking in another's shoes is not easy, you have to try to step into them. At that point, the question becomes: Now, how would I want to be treated?
- You can also try just a simple smile and acknowledgment. The power of your face could shock you. It creates other smiles, and instantly bring down walls.

- Think of a time when you were excluded. Perhaps it was back in high school or at a party where everyone else was having fun or at the water cooler at work. How did it feel to be on the outside? Once you let that feeling back into your heart, you'll stop seeing differences as barriers.
- Think about the steps it took for the person you feel like judging to reach where they are today. Was it easy? Now think of the steps it took you to get to where you are. While we all need courage to overcome challenges, some climbs are steeper than others. In addition to empathy and compassion, don't be afraid to let admiration for others develop.
- Remember that people enter your life for a reason and each meeting is an opportunity. Open your mind to the lesson that each person can teach you about life and about yourself.

LESSON 8

Follow Your Heart and Others Will Too

You may say I'm a dreamer. But I'm not the only one.

– John Lennon

Vulnerability is often given a bad rap. It's known as a sign of weakness when really, it's anything but. Losing that mask, and revealing yourself to the world, does expose you—in the best possible way. When you allow others to see the real person you are inside, there's no doubt about it: That's you demonstrating great strength.

Due to Jacob's vulnerability, he attracts many. He can't hide his true nature, like most of us do in our everyday lives. This openness, which comes to him naturally, is called following your heart. And I have learned that when I follow my heart, I rarely have regrets.

I have also learned that when you truly follow your heart, others will follow theirs, as well.

After Jacob's initial diagnosis, Jeff and I couldn't bear the thought of other families going through the same heartache. We were vulnerable and our hearts were telling us that we needed to share

our experience with others. We couldn't allow other families to be
blindsided, to have to find their way through the pain without help.
So we came out of the closet, so to speak. We stood up and told
our story and our family, friends and community rallied together.

That's how our grassroots charity, Jacob's Ladder, was born.

Officially named the Canadian Foundation for the Control of
Neurodegenerative Disease, Jacob's Ladder is a non-profit organization
that funds research, education, awareness and therapy into neurodegenerative illnesses. I'm proud to say that as of today, Jacob's
Ladder has raised more than $2.5 million and has saved countless
lives. As a direct result of our initiatives, parents across Canada can
be screened for Canavan Disease at no cost and without hassle. It
is now possible to tell, with more than 95 percent certainty, whether
one or both parents is a carrier of the disease. Complete strangers
on the street will often hug me followed by a whisper of gratitude
for the information that is now accessible to them.

And that was just the beginning. Once we realized that Jacob's
Ladder could make great strides in helping people with special
needs, and that giving creates a ripple effect, we kept going. Our
mission was and still is not just to find creative ways to give, but
to mobilize our community to join us.

We fund an international award, the Norman Saunders Award
in Genetics, at the Hospital for Sick Children in Toronto. Norm
Saunders was Jacob's first pediatrician and our close friend. He
helped us to navigate through the complicated hospital system, in
the aptly named area of complex care. He was a dear friend, a
mentor to so many and a model pediatrician who was ahead of his

time when it comes to patient care. Sadly, Norman Saunders passed away but this award lives on as a legacy to his dedication, warmth and brilliance.

Norman believed in doctors and researchers collaborating together, and in honor of that tradition, our prize is awarded each year to a doctor who has made great strides in research and discovery. The winner comes to Toronto to share their findings with our pediatricians at the Hospital for Sick Children. So far, honorees have come from the likes of Baylor College of Medicine in Texas, Harvard University, Johns Hopkins University, The University of Edinburgh and Oxford University.

Norman Saunders followed his heart and we followed his lead. We were thrilled by the screening, the funded research studies and the annual international award, but it wasn't enough. We knew that Jacob's life was going to be short, we wanted him to always be remembered. And so we began searching for a legacy project to honor Jacob and his life. For years, we racked our brains to find just the right project. We wanted a bricks and mortar project, something we could touch and feel, something that would resonate not just with our Jacob but with so many disabled kids in our world. And then we found the perfect project.

Jacob loves to swim. Once submerged into warm water, his limbs relax, allowing his body to float to the surface. As I hold his head above the water, I see an expression of ecstasy. It is right here that my child feels alive and free.

The water is such a beautiful gift that we were determined to share it. Because so many people can benefit from the magic of water therapy, we funded the Jacob's Ladder Therapeutic Pool, which was opened in 2012. This massive pool, situated in the state-of-the-art Schwartz/Reisman Centre north of Toronto, welcomes everyone who might need it to access water therapy.

As Jacob grows older, we notice more and more ways that people in our community are desperately in need of help. One woefully underfunded and overlooked area is programming for adults with special needs. In fact, when students hit the age of 21, all funded programming in Ontario abruptly comes to an end. What are parents to do? What are these young adults to do when they no longer have a support network that provides a sense of belonging and purpose? One day, their lives are stimulated and full and then next, they are dragged down by long wait-list times, limited opportunities and hefty fees for service.

At Jacob's Ladder, this is one area of great need that merits our attention and research. We are finding ways to help subsidize some of this funding that can open some doors for young adults who find themselves in this very bleak, much underfunded chasm.

None of these goals could have been reached by our efforts alone. Yes, we started by following our hearts, but it wasn't until our community backed us that the initiatives took flight. Our supporters were right there with us from the get go. They helped plan, helped raise funds, spread the word, made it happen. From our first silent auction at our local Starbucks, to our golf tournaments, to our movie nights, to our raffles, to our Family Fun Days, to our concerts, our community was out in full force. The ripple effect is real. As Helen Keller stated, "Alone we can do so little, together we can do so much."

Are you in tune with your purpose, your passion, your mission? Wondering how you can help make a difference in the world? Here are some ideas for how you can open your heart to the possibilities and make the world a richer place.

- Think about what you really want to do. What moves you? No matter how difficult it seems, allow yourself the freedom to envision it. Then go for it!
- Asking for support from others is key so don't be shy. Keep this motto in mind: If you don't ask, you don't get.
- Be prepared for, and okay, with the answer "no." Do people say no sometimes? Of course they do. Does it sting? Sometimes. But that's okay. The "yes" is worth the risk.
- Consider what matters to you in life, and what you think might make the world a better place. Start spreading it around.
- Research community efforts and see if any strike you. Volunteer to get on board.
- Get creative with friends. Just because you're not sure how to turn your idea into a reality doesn't mean it can't be done. Brainstorm and see what you come up with together.

LESSON 9

Believe in Your Vision

You miss 100% of the shots you don't take.

— Wayne Gretzky

I am an ideas person. Ideas continuously come and go in my head. Once in a while, a vision will appear and it just won't leave. All I need to make it happen in real life is a little shove. Years ago, I had another of my big ideas while lying in bed. I looked over at Jeff and shared it. "I'm going to write a book." He looked at me with a loving smile and said, "I'll believe that when I see it."

And there it was—my shove. I jumped out of bed, ran to my computer and started to type. One year later, *Lessons from Jacob: A Disabled Son Teaches his Mother About Courage, Hope and the Joy of Living Each Day to the Fullest* was on bookstore shelves. And now, here we go again.

One of the most beautiful things about raising funds for Jacob's Ladder is creating a vision. What follows is beautiful too—working with passionate people to develop, foster and turn that vision into an actual event.

Our first event to kick off Jacob's Ladder was an evening hosted by our local Starbucks. They rallied the other stores in our neighborhood to donate items for a silent auction. There was free coffee, mingling with neighbors and local entertainment all set up at our Starbucks. From there, we were on a roll. Next came a movie night, followed by a golf tournament. And then the inevitable big idea struck: Family Fun Day filled with teachable moments.

As parents of young children, we were always searching for activities to do as a family, especially on weekends. As Jacob is at our family's core, we wanted Jacob's Ladder to revolve around family fun that kids can enjoy.

Our Family Fun Day vision came alive in our family room, where all planning takes place. When we are coming up with ideas, our muse, Jacob, is always right there in the center of the room since he is our cause, our inspiration. He lies on his oversized ottoman, literally right in the heart of the meeting.

Our newest incarnation of Family Fun Days is called Jake's Gigantic Give and it's based on the feelings associated with giving. With small budgets in place, we called on family and friends to help plan the weekend event. It's a time for everyone to get in on the giving spirit—the guests, the committee, the volunteers, the vendors, the performers and the sponsors, everyone.

Our first Jake's Gigantic Give taught us so much about how to fulfill our vision. First, we needed a venue where we could transform an empty space into a lavish toy store. We had arranged to collect more than 85 skids of donated toys from Mastermind Toys, Spinmaster Toys and The Canadian Group so we needed a large enough space and to be able to borrow it for weeks. We put the word out and our friends came through. They had an empty store in Toronto that they generously lent us, free of charge.

For weeks, after school and on weekends, our committee members met at our venue with children of all ages. We carefully unpacked hundreds of boxes filled with the latest toys. It was a children's paradise. Games, scooters, remote-control cars, dolls, stuffed animals and a random assortment of toys for all ages were everywhere.

Our friends put their lives on hold to devote time and energy to help create a magical setting for Jake's Gigantic Give. Staging companies lent us décor. A slew of carpets, modern furniture, fixtures and coffee tables were delivered and distributed to create a funky club-like lounge. And there was more. Westbury Entertainment unloaded a truck filled with sound equipment, drapery, staging, lights and television screens and dozens of their employees donated their own time to help us set up.

The food vendors were all in place to hand out free food. The entertainers were all set to fuel souls with their magical voices. The volunteers in our store were all lined up to greet guests. Hundreds of teenaged volunteers were dressed in blue t-shirts with angel wings on their backs. They could hardly wait to take children on their tour.

Finally, we were ready. Jake's Gigantic Give was about to happen. The doors opened and guests arrived at the grand entrance. Each angel volunteer guided a family on a remarkable journey where they chose gifts to give to others just in time for the holidays.

Parents had the choice to join their children on this adventure or to hang out in the Jacob's Ladder lounge where they could eat, drink and socialize with friends over a free sampling of delicious snacks and Starbucks coffee.

While parents were occupied, their kids were guided through an inspirational tour led by a teen angel, who took the time to sit with each young guest to review their personal mission card.

Together, they read:

> TODAY YOU WILL MAKE ANOTHER CHILD SMILE
> THE TRUE GIFT IS THE ONE THAT YOU GIVE AWAY

> Some questions for you to consider.
> Do you get to eat three meals a day?
> Do you sleep in a bed?
> Do you feel good today?
> Do you ever get presents for holidays or birthdays?
> Does someone love you very much?

> Our guess is you said, "Yes."
> Many children would answer, "No."
> Your mission is to brighten a child's day.
> Yes, you can make a difference today.

> Imagine a child similar in age to you.
> A boy or a girl? What do they like to do?
> Think of this special person whose spirits you will lift.

> Imagine what this person may like and then find the
> perfect gift.

And off they went, carrying an empty bag in their hands, which would soon be overflowing with gifts. First, they entered a store where nothing can be purchased, only given away. With jaws dropped, children roamed the premises with their mission in mind to create a beautiful gift for a child in need.

Next, the kids were led to a wrapping station where they could wrap the gifts they had collected and design a homemade card for their lucky recipient. Since many toys were too large for small hands, their angel would then carry the homemade gift to an area where representatives from five different charities were on hand to receive it and explain who would get to open it over the holidays. No matter the child's age, by now, that magical sensation of giving to others was already a part of them.

Just before the children were to reunite with their parents, each charity representative took a moment to present a gift card from Jacob. The card entitled each child to choose one toy to keep. It was a small token of appreciation for a huge act of kindness, but interestingly, many children wanted to keep on giving. Without much thought, they handed over their gift to charity as well.

As families reunited after their mission, they gathered in Jake's Lounge to enjoy free concerts by talented young performers.

Because giving was the theme of this event, everything imaginable was donated. It wasn't about the value of the gifts in terms of dollars; it was about the community banding together in a purely selfless manner.

We were in awe of the hundreds who believed in our vision, and so, to thank everyone for their selflessness, we wrote this letter on Jacob's behalf.

> Look what we did together! Hundreds came to discover magic, *Pure Magic*. All of you helped in your own unique and powerful way. Thousands of gifts were given away to those who need them most. Hundreds of teenagers were role models leading youngsters on a mission of kindness. This weekend showcased the contagious and heartfelt power that we all have in us to give unconditionally and unselfishly.

> Look what people are saying...

> My kids learned a valuable lesson about giving to others.

> Incredibly Inspiring.

> Maddy went to bed in her angel shirt as she said it made her "feel good."

> Jack felt so proud of himself and his brothers for donating gifts to others. As he was going to bed tonight, Jack said that he was proud of his little brother's good deed. I think that is pretty special coming from a four-year-old boy.

Thank you to all of you for being part of the Jacob's Ladder family. As we take a moment to pause and reflect, an overwhelming feeling of calm and comfort takes over. We are completely humbled by this community. At first, you were there for us. Now all of us are there for so many others.

From everything we have in us, we wish to thank all of you for helping to drive this vision. From our family to yours: Look what we have *All Done Together!*

With Love and great appreciation,

Jacob and his family

Jake's life has been one massive Jake's Gigantic Give, and Jacob is the best gift of all. So how can we give? How can we make something out of nothing? How can we all make a difference? Here are some ideas that may inspire you.

- If you've got a vision you want to turn into a reality, consider what steps you'll need to take. Once you start creating, others will feel your passion and join your team.
- Surround yourselves with like-minded people who will be willing to help crystallize your vision. So much can come out of positive energy. It's infectious, so let people into the circle to help it grow.
- Be prepared to give all that you have to give, especially if you've got others on board to help. If you put your whole heart into everything that you do, they will, too.

- Find people you admire and work closely with them. The best results come from working with people you respect.
- Taking the lead is fine but always be prepared to actively listen and be open to new ideas and different perspectives.
- Don't think about what's in it for you; think about what you are doing for others. Believe me, when you are focused on helping others, you will help yourself in ways you never even imagined.

LESSON 10

Be Grateful,
Take The Jake Challenge

"What day is it?" asked Pooh.
"It's today," squealed Piglet.
"My favourite day," said Pooh.

– A. A. Milne

Every day is a blessing. Every year Jacob is with us is a miracle. How does he do it? What makes him tick and keep on ticking? How does he continue to fight each day with everything he has in him? He is such an inspiration that on Jake's 15th birthday, our family took a quiet challenge to honor his life. Thinking about the challenges he faces every day, we tried to figure out his secret. How can he be so positive with so many odds stacked against him? Here's what we came up with.

Jacob instinctively and naturally follows three rules in life:

    1. Always be positive.

2. Always appreciate everyone and everything that surrounds you.
3. Always live each moment to the fullest.

Of course, it's great advice for anyone. But the reality is, these three simple rules are much easier to say than to live by. We know because we put ourselves to the test. I tried to live like Jake, and guess what happened. I failed.

I set out to see the world in a positive light and to appreciate every moment, but within minutes, negative thoughts fought their way into my brain. As soon as my own expectations for how the day should unfold went unfulfilled, disappointment set in and I could feel myself getting all frustrated and judgmental. But having those rules in the back of my mind did help. It created a frame of perspective within which I could make a conscious effort to let go of my judgments and hone in on a more positive approach.

Specifically, I worked on shifting my point of view when it comes to how other people act. While I couldn't change the actions of others, I realized that what I could change was my reaction to them. Now, instead of feeling hurt or disappointed, I told myself that those actions are the direct result of whatever the person went through earlier that day. That "empathy shift" allowed me to switch my thinking from negative to positive because it freed me from the equation and, once free, I could focus on feeling appreciative again.

Gratitude is something that comes naturally to Jacob and, lucky for me, I get a front row seat to watch how it works in action. I let his appreciation for the little things in life give me perspective. He expects nothing and is therefore always surprised by what he receives. I try to follow his lead.

Most people don't realize just how far a little old-fashioned appreciation goes in relationships. When my mother is at a doctor's appointment, she jots down notes in her pad. She's not reminding herself of the complicated instructions she has to follow. Rather, she's making notes so she can return at a later date with gifts in hand to thank the medical staff for taking the time to help.

My parents are experts at appreciation. They make it a point to give gifts to anyone who has helped them. Whether it's the gas station attendant, the waitress at their favorite restaurant, the gentleman who shines my father's shoes, the golf caddy or a doctor or nurse, everyone deserves gratitude. If people are kind to my parents, my parents are even kinder back.

I can't count how many times I've heard these words: "Oh my gosh, they are your parents? They are the most generous people I know." And as a result, their lives are even fuller. Everywhere they go, people go out of their way to make their lives easier.

Like my parents, Jacob is always appreciative of the kindness that others show him. Although he can't show his feelings through words or thoughtful gestures of thanks, he demonstrates it in the only way that he knows how—in his smile.

Interestingly, gratitude is also a selfish act—in the best possible way. When you are grateful, you are happier. Longing for the greener grass makes you feel perpetually unsatisfied, but grateful-ness brings a feeling of satisfaction like none other.

To celebrate Jacob's 16th birthday, we wanted to share this new perspective. I called three girlfriends, told them about the three rules and asked them to join the challenge. To help others get on board, we designed a bracelet to get everyone started. Right there on our wrists would be all the reminder we needed to redefine our priorities, to view life just like Jake, to help us slow down and focus on what truly matters.

After exploring one bead boutique after another, we found what we were after and created a unique bracelet of inspiration. It is the centerpiece in what we call The Jake Challenge. I like to think of this piece of jewelry as a physical moral compass to conceptualize the challenge to give thanks. At the same time, it is a symbol of a remarkable life, so well-lived despite its challenges. We made 300 beautiful bracelets in honor of Jake's 16th birthday.

Each bracelet came with the following instructions:

Against all odds, Jacob is able to live life to the fullest.

For many miraculous years, he has followed these three simple rules.

He appreciates everything and everyone.

He lives in the moment.

He's so positive.

Here's how the bracelet works. Turn the shiny bead toward your heart every time you find yourself following Jake's rules. If you slip, turn the bead away from your heart. Seem simple? Give it a try and take the challenge!

I know when I follow Jake's lead, my day is a whole lot brighter.

Love Ellen

Through word of mouth alone, The Jake Challenge bracelets became an instant hit. They were sold out in 24 hours. So we made another 300 and, again, we were sold out in a day. That's when we called in the troops. Our friends, family and many, many children came together to bead away to great tunes, goodies and treats.

Whenever I receive an order for more bracelets or bump into someone wearing the bracelet, I am overcome by joy. One summer day, I received a call from a friend who placed an order. That night, I got to work. Sixteen bracelets coming up, plus one male Jake Challenge bracelet as a gift for my friend who graciously ordered so many.

After I shipped off the package, I received an e-mail from him. "Ellen, I think there is a problem with the order." I couldn't imagine what went wrong. I had carefully counted 16 bracelets, each with dark brown beads and one shiny bead.

He explained. "What I really want is for all of them to look like the one that you made for me." What I failed to realize was that he was ordering 16 male bracelets. I was so used to women's orders that my design was all wrong.

And then came the kicker. The bracelets weren't for his friends at all. "Ellen, they are all for me!" my friend explained. "I need backup because if a bracelet breaks or I forget to put it on one morning, I want to make sure I always have extras on hand."

This man's dedication to gratitude in his life is part of what fuels mine to challenge others to do so. As we turn our beads towards our hearts, we are grateful for Jacob's three rules, for Jacob, our family, our network of friends and our sensational community. And there's an unexpected bonus. Since the inauguration of The Jake Challenge in 2013, our little project has raised more than $30,000, and counting, for research, awareness and education into neuro-degenerative illnesses.

How can we stop now? Each night, after dinner, we continue to bead with a smile. It's part of our life now—to make beautiful things, to challenge others to live their best life, to better the world.

Gratefulness takes some work. How do we turn negative thoughts into positive ones? You can do it consciously, by taking these steps.

- Before you react, always ask yourself: Why is this person acting this way? You may think you know the answer, but you might not. Try to give them the benefit of doubt.
- Instead of feeling drawn into other people's negativity, be an open ear. Listen to what they are complaining about and do some nodding. Just by helping them feel understood and heard, you are creating positive energy.
- When you find yourself in a situation with someone who is truly negative, use it as a trigger to be grateful for the people who you choose to surround yourself with.

- Remember, we cannot change others. We can only change how we react when we find ourselves in negative situations. Use this to rise up and turn your own thoughts around.
- If you shy away from negative people, then be attuned to your negativity as well.
- If you find someone being rude to you, try to be kind before extricating yourself. Often, a simple act of kindness will turn a situation around.

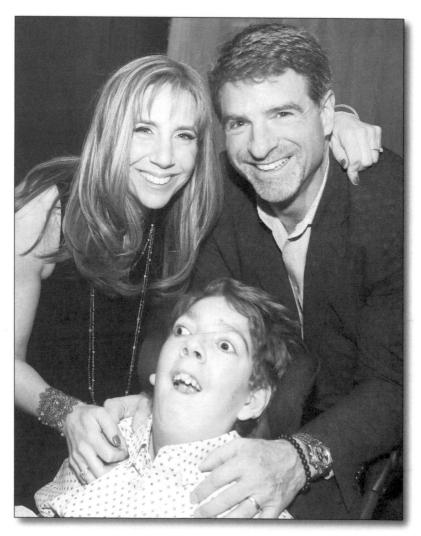

Jake with Ellen and Jeff

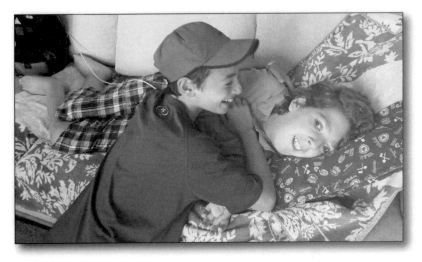

Ben with Jacob

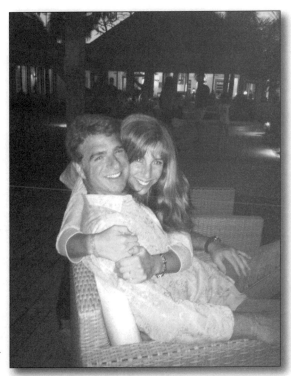

Ellen and Jeff

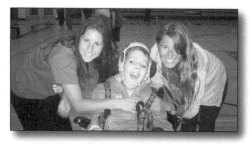

Jake at Bayview Glen Day Camp
with Aly and Danielle

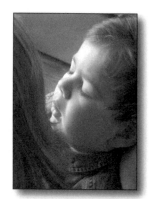

Jacob at three years old

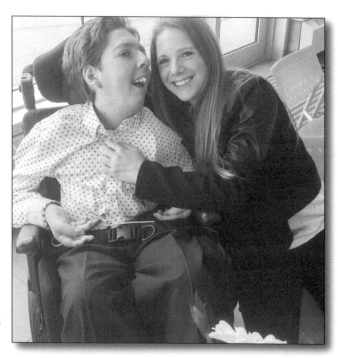

Jake with his
sister Bevvy

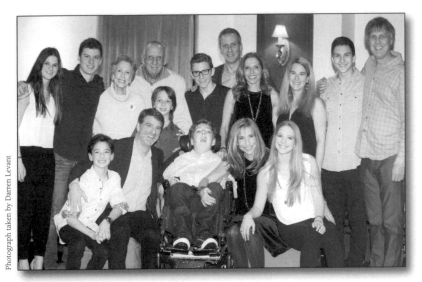

Levy Family

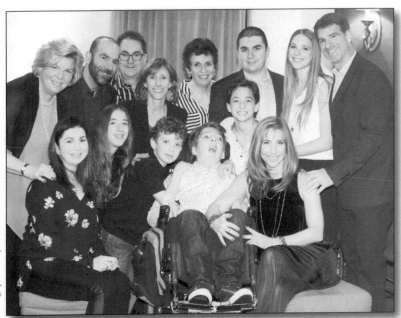

Schwartz Family

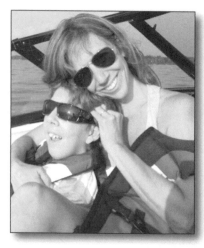

Jake boating
with Ellen

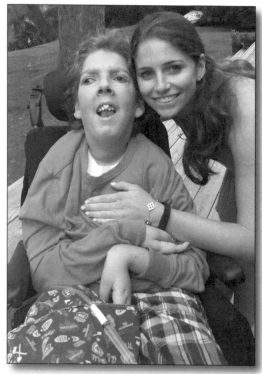

Jacob with Ali Goodbaum

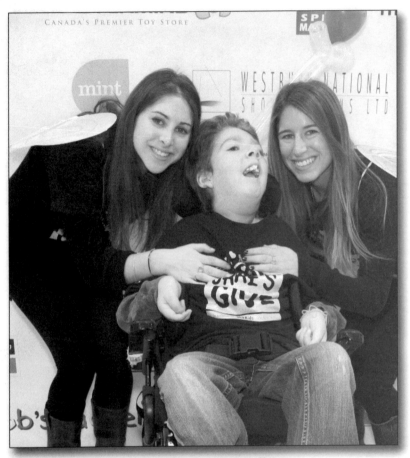

Jake with his Bayview Glen Angels, Aly and Danielle

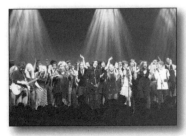

Jake's Jam – The Finale

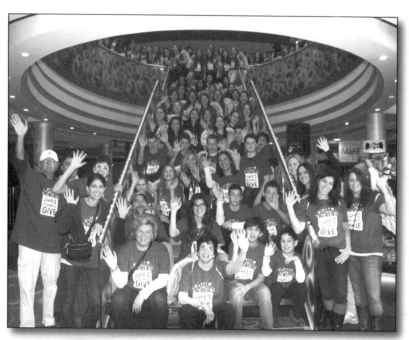

Volunteers at Jake's Gigantic Give

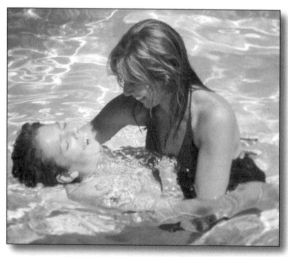

Jake swimming
with Ellen

LESSON 11

Memorize the Moment

God gave us memory so that we might have roses in December.

— J.M. Barrie

We come across them all the time but we don't always notice. They are these perfect Kodak moments, when you are very far from your camera or phone but you need to take that shot. You absolutely must freeze this moment so you can bank it and access it whenever you need to. Do yourself the most beautiful favor. Next time you find yourself in what you would call a moment of bliss, connect with your senses—stop, listen, look, smell, touch, feel. Memorize every part of the moment.

When I'm up north, these moments seem to keep coming. The day starts early. While everyone is still asleep, I pour my coffee and take it down to the dock. I sit and listen to the waves crashing against the rocks, feeling the breeze off the lake and the morning sun kissing my skin. I sip to the chorus of birdsong. I shut my eyes. I am memorizing the moment.

Like most people, I am pulled in every direction during the week, and when that happens, my memorized moments bring me peace. All I have to do is shut my eyes and I find it—a little breath of weekend air to save me from the chaos.

Jacob lives inside every moment. He is perpetually in the here and now. How brilliant! Most of us are so busy recounting what just happened or so lost in worry over what will happen next that we miss what's going on right now. Not Jacob. He is only focused on each moment as it unfolds. Wouldn't it be amazing if we could all capture every moment of bliss?

Jake and I recently enjoyed a night out at the theater. I wheeled his chair onto the plush carpet at the elegant Princess of Wales Theatre in Toronto and locked it into place at the back of the Orchestra section. I pulled up the red velvet chair right beside so I could put my arm behind his shoulders and lean in close. Patrons in the last row of connected seats twisted around to check out the person behind them whose breathing was labored.

They saw me. I was nervous because I didn't want Jake's experience at the play to ruin anyone else's and I knew all too well what was coming. Sometimes, when he's excited, Jacob vocalizes his enthusiasm. It sometimes explodes at quiet moments. With these strangers' eyes on me, I needed to communicate many things at once: My discomfort, my empathy, a plea for understanding. So I acknowledged them with a smile and a nod. I tipped my head down toward Jacob, giving each person's face my gaze, one by one. I hoped that they would interpret my smile to mean, I'm sorry if my son gets loud during the production. When they nodded and smiled back, I was grateful. Message received.

The house lights dimmed and the orchestra began to play. I peered over at Jacob and watched his eyes and mouth radiate joy. I squeezed him to acknowledge the moment we were sharing. As he absorbed every second of the first act, I closed my eyes to memorize this moment. In his glory, Jacob reveled in the live performance while I', in mine, reveled at my son. He was center stage for me. I marveled at his giggle, his excitable breathing, the elegant ambiance surrounding us, the velvety hug of the chair and the happiness of his features. There is no greater joy than witnessing someone you love feel joy.

The play lasted for two and a half hours, but the intensity of that moment I experienced with Jacob will last forever.

When we find ourselves in blissful moments, we have to take the time to take a mental snapshot of it. Look carefully and study everything about this brief moment in time until you can close your eyes and see it. If you do it right, you'll always be able to bring that moment back when you need it most.

To celebrate two milestones in our lives, Jake's tenth birthday and my fortieth, Jeff and I decided to plan a family trip to Disney World. Not an easy feat with healthy children. Now imagine throwing a medically challenged child into the mix. For weeks, Jeff spent hours on the telephone with Air Canada to secure a safe flight for our family. This included preparations to take all precautions necessary. We needed to travel with Jacob's numerous amounts of medication, his food pump, his suction machine as well as all chargers and back up chargers. As Jacob cannot sit upright and wheelchairs are not permitted on airplanes, Jeff arranged for an empty seat behind Jacob's seat as it had to be reclined to its maximum capacity.

Once Jeff and I carried Jacob down the narrow aisle of the airplane and settled him into his seat, we stuffed a dozen or so pillows all around him to secure his position. Finally, Jacob was all prepped, ready to go. Now it was time to settle our eight-year-old Bevvy and our four-year-old Ben. We did it! We made it to Orlando and we were so thrilled that we did.

Getting there was a marathon of sorts, but no one does special needs like Disney. Everything is wheelchair accessible and they bend over backwards to help in any way possible. This includes entering the rides by the exits and staying on them as long as the children wish. At Disney, Jake had rock star status in the minds of Bev and Ben.

Anyone who has small children understands all too well the hustle and bustle of getting youngsters dressed, sun screened, hydrated and ready for a day on vacation. On this trip, our daily routine consisted of swimming in the hotel pool in the morning, having lunch and then packing up for an afternoon at Magic Kingdom.

One day, after lunch, Jeff was in the hotel room dressing Jacob and collecting all of his medication and supplies for our four-hour excursion. It was my job to get the other two kids ready to go and, clearly, rushing was not on their agenda. They were playing in the sand. Bevvy, was giving her younger brother a piggy back ride. They kept falling down and belly laughing as I tried to hurry them along so we could move forward with our plans.

I grabbed Ben by the hand and started to walk with him. Bev didn't follow. She just stood there, bare feet in the sand, blond hair blowing in the breeze, her belly bulging from her pink bikini. She was gazing at the magnificent pool right beside her, complete with fountains, waterfalls and rock staircases.

"Bev." No answer. I called louder. "Bevvy!" Louder. "Beverly, let's go!" Now I was shouting.

She turned around and staring straight at me, she said, "Mom, I'm memorizing the moment!"

She knew that this moment was a chance of a lifetime. She didn't want to let it pass so fast. She knew that we can't always go to Florida, but if needed, we can bring that sunshine paradise home to us.

And then there was Italy, a surprise and delight that changed my life. In the book *Lessons from Jacob*, I shared an analogy about life with a child with disabilities written by a writer from *Sesame Street*, Emily Perl Kingsley. It was about a family planning a trip of a lifetime to Italy. What happens instead is that their plane takes a turn and lands in Holland. So what do they do? They learn to face the fact that they may not get to Italy and they go on to discover all of the beauty Holland has to offer. Years ago, after Jake's diagnosis, I found a photocopy of this analogy in my mailbox. To this day, I don't know who left it there, but I am forever grateful.

The irony of receiving this anonymous gift was that it was just the kick we needed to fulfill our lifelong dream of traveling to Italy. Jeff and I finally made it come true to commemorate our 20th anniversary. Even though I had never been, I could already taste the freshness of the ripe tomatoes plucked from vines and smell the fragrance of lemon trees. I had always dreamed of being greeted by the open-hearted passionate Italian people and now I would.

Of course, there was work to do, and lots of it. A trip overseas, which we were taking with two other couples, requires hours upon hours of planning, searching, investigating and dreaming. Everyone was giddy with excitement. Except secretly, I was scared. My stomach felt sick at the very thought of leaving Jacob. The feeling was overwhelming, and every day I fought it until my insides felt bruised as a punching bag. I so wanted to go, but my heart wasn't letting me want.

I was tethered by questions. How could I go so far away? How would Jacob do without me checking in regularly? Could I really separate from him? What if he needed me? What if I needed him? The guilt, anguish, contemplation and excitement of going on this trip was almost too much to bear. *Almost.*

We left Jake in extraordinary hands. On the kitchen bulletin board, there was a color-coded mess of arrangements we had planned for Jacob in our absence. There was backup planned for backup. Each day, he was picked up by two special educators, who took him on outings. When he wasn't exploring the city with them, he was at home with two caregivers who loved him like their own. While his brother and sister were off at camp, he was surrounded by his favorite people and visited by family members daily. Off we went.

Scenes from movies, photographs online and pretty postcards cannot do justice to this breathtaking land on earth. Everywhere you look, it is picture perfect. If ever there was a moment to memorize, it was our time in the Aeolian Islands, off the coast of Sicily.

Bougainvillea line streets that climb up and down mountains. Crystal blue waters wrap around volcanic islands. There are beaches of black ash sands created from falling volcanic pebbles. The menus are based on fresh produce picked right from the islands. We enjoyed capers, almonds, citrus and homemade wine from the rows and rows of vineyards rising up the mountains from the sea. A head turn to the left, mountains, a head turn to the right, the sea.

The trip was monumental in so many ways, but there is one mental snapshot that always takes me back.

The six of us spent the day out on the open sea in a small cruising boat built for twelve. There were three rows of white vinyl seats that reclined all the way back into beds. Jeff and I took ownership of the third row. Our guide brought snacks, water and wine. We were all set for the tour of a lifetime. With music blasting and friends sharing this journey, we set out to hop from one island to the next. The cooling breeze against my hot skin and the purr of the motor would have been memorable enough, but then a feeling of freedom overcame me. On a calm sunny day, we were in the middle of the sea, with nothing but exploration ahead.

The activities kept us immersed in nature. One moment we were snorkeling in a clear blue cove, and the next we were exploring an island and sitting down in a local pizzeria in just-wet bathing suits and cover-ups.

The hours vanished like seconds and before we knew it, our guide said it was getting late and we had better get back to our boat before dark. As we drove away from the island of Stromboli, all covered in soot and black ash, we could see the sun dropping. We anchored our boat and sat together drinking wine and watching the colors of yellow, orange and red as they blended in the evening sky.

When darkness fell, we waited and waited, never wanting to leave. Suddenly, we heard a strange loud crumbling sound. We watched Stromboli come alive as the fire resting inside the belly of the active volcano released its lava and it bubbled over the side of the mountain. We heard the rumble of burning rocks as they fell, sizzling as they hit the sea.

We were wide-eyed, all of our senses on alert. We couldn't believe what we were witnessing. Too late, we grabbed our cameras and our phones to try to freeze the moment. But it couldn't be captured on film. It could only live in our memories.

That evening, we coasted back to our island. The night was dark but illuminated by millions of stars overhead. Jeff and I snuggled up as the chill set in. All I could hear was the buzz of the motor and the water splashing against the side of our boat. The moment was perfectly ours, and one that could never be replicated. Just after Jeff was lulled to sleep by the hum of the motor, I sobbed and sobbed.

Were these tears of sadness? I don't think so. Were they tears of joy? Not sure. What I do know is that the moment was raw and beautiful enough to let in and experience deeply. With no filter blocking me, I was able to just let go of whatever was holding me back. Now, whenever I need to release, I go straight back to that boat on the Aeolian Islands in my mind, and I feel free.

How do we manage to capture the most valuable moments in life so we can relive them again and again? Chances are, you can't always go back to that happy place, but if you memorize the moment, you can recall the experience on demand.

- The most important thing is to be connected to how you feel. If you find yourself in a state of calmness or joy, focus on that feeling. Turn it over in your mind and body. Don't let it go so quickly.
- Close your eyes and listen to the sounds around you. Physically take notice of the wind or air brushing against your skin. What is that smell?
- Work all of your senses, one at a time, to capture all of the experience.
- Take in the moment consciously and lock it into your memory bank.
- Watch and feel the moment over and over. Continue to reel it in throughout that day and evening. Yes, this takes practice.
- Remember that once your moment has been captured, it will be ready for you to retrieve whenever you need it. Give it a try!

LESSON 12

Worry Time

Worry does not empty tomorrow of its sorrow,
it empties today of its strength.

– Corrie ten Boom

Parents worry. It's just what we do, and it's something we're expert at—for good reason. From the time our children are born, there's so much worry involved, it can make us nuts, and it just grows along with them. Are they eating enough? Are they eating too much? Am I being too strict? Am I being too lenient? Where are they now? What are they doing? Are they okay? Are they happy?

Here's a saying that speaks to so many of us: As a parent, you are only as happy as your saddest child. That about sums it up.

In life in general, I have always considered myself a professional worrier. So when I was faced with a child who was born with something to really worry about, that's all I did. Worrying compounded the problem in ways I couldn't measure. I was savvy enough to know, though, that what I was doing wasn't healthy for me and it certainly wasn't helping Jacob.

Worry can debilitate you. If there's too much of it, it can interfere with function. That's why, early on, I learned to compartmentalize it. Worry was taking up prime real estate in my head, and it needed to be evicted—or at least moved—so I could be productive.

What did I do? I created a particular time of day that would be dedicated to worry. Usually, it's just for ten minutes. For me, it's shower time. While I'm washing the rest of me, I allow myself a bonus. I cleanse not only my body, but my thoughts and emotions, too. Then comes the next step. Right after the shower, I control as many of the worries as I can by addressing all problems that are fixable. I pen that list, I send that pending e-mail, I make those phone calls, I complete whichever tasks were making me worry so the emotions associated with them will abate.

If what I'm worried about cannot be solved because it's out of my control, then worrying about it all day will do nothing but make me feel worse. But it's not as if we can just push a button to make the emotion disappear. So I do something about it. I say to myself, "Ellen you have worried about this, long and hard. There is nothing you can do at this time. Worry about it later."

And I follow my own advice. I force myself to delay until I'm in the right headspace. I wait until Worry Time comes around the next day, when I've carved out specific time that is dedicated to worry.

This neat little trick has been a life saver. Although it does take time to master, it improves the day. Soon, Worry Time will become a habit. Now, compartmentalizing worry into its own time frame works well when life is rolling along in a steady routine. But, when life gets hard, really hard, almost impossible, there may be too much worry to contain. In that case, you may need some other tactics.

I did some research. I asked more than a hundred friends and family members who have experienced tragedy, "What exactly helped you to get through the worst times?" The answers were filled with some amazing techniques that can help you to lower the worry quotient and survive even the heaviest stress. I notice that these responses fit into six distinct categories: Me Time, Meditation, Family and Friends, Self-Reflection, Gratitude and Gaining Perspective, Finding an Outlet and Regaining Normalcy. Here are their responses.

Take Me Time
- Be quiet by yourself, with time to figure it out; be sad or angry or whatever the emotion of the day is.
- Put it all into perspective and then get on with it.
- Make alone time for you and your spouse. Stressful times can make you feel all alone and cause tension. Feeling the reconnection helps.

Use Meditation
- Do a relaxation body scan. It is a guided meditation where you focus your attention and your breath on successive body parts starting from your toes and continuing until you reach your head. The combination

of slowing your breathing and focusing on feeling your
toes, belly, shoulders and so on allows a brief break from
the endless stewing loop in your brain.

- Become aware of your breathing and of letting go.
- Be in the moment, whether that's in a seated meditation
  or a walking one.
- Use mindfulness apps to help your brain calm down/turn
  off so you can sleep.

Lean on Loved Ones

- Talk through your anxieties and fears with someone who
  is sympathetic, encouraging and knowledgeable about
  what you are going through. This person needs to be a
  good listener, someone who will let you vent and will
  give you a realistic perspective.
- Plan something to look forward to, like a day trip or a
  getaway with your spouse, kids or friends. It's so
  important to have something to look forward to.
- Confide in a friend or loved one and express yourself
  openly and honestly. Talking aloud is very helpful and
  builds strength and trust.
- Give yourself permission to find humor, even if it is black
  humor, in the darkest moments.
- Allow those closest to you to help. Say yes to offers of
  assistance when other times you take care of things
  yourself.

- Be open to talking to those you trust and feel close to about your experiences and feelings. This may be hard for guys who think they are supposed to tough it out, even in traumatic life situations. Avoiding discussions around painful topics tends to make them worse while opening up can feel like a relief.

Engage in Reflection
- Remember that things change.
- Look at old photos and positive reminders/memories of happy times.
- Immerse yourself in wisdom/biblical study to refresh your thinking and reset your perspective.
- Go for a walk and talk to God. He's always available and is a great listener, and if you listen from your soul, you may even perceive a response.
- Write your feelings down about the person who is suffering.
- Go to a support group. Sharing experiences and supporting others facing similar loss is both cathartic and helpful.
- Never give up by focusing on what is really important in life. Stay strong and healthy, if not for yourself, then for your loved ones.
- Pray, even if you aren't used to praying. It's a good time to start.
- Have the solid belief that things will get better somehow, some way.

- Seek professional help. Doing so will help you understand what you're going through right now and what's coming next. It will help to organize your thoughts and worries.
- Create a Sabbath, whether that's one day a week, an hour every day or even a few minutes periodically. There has to be a respite from what is a time-driven struggle to keep up with demands imposed on us (or self-imposed). A true Sabbath is not just a rest. It is an embrace of the spirit, the spark that enlivens us. It is a time beyond time. If you can find that kind of respite, you are blessed, for during that period, an ordering of priorities takes place, and you return to the world with a more robust triage system. More importantly, you get a glimpse into your place in the universe and an intuition that you are a part of something vast and perhaps noble.
- Surrender. Recognize that this is a difficult time and it will likely pass.
- Find strength in solitude. There, you'll be infused with the energy you need to move forward.
- Remind yourself that this too shall pass. Remember that you have endured other very difficult times and made it despite believing you wouldn't at the time.
- Eat without reading or watching television. Drive without listening to music or talking on the phone. Try to be present wherever you are.

- Sit in a dark room, take a number of deep breaths and try to deconstruct why you are feeling stress. Then consider what you can do to relieve it.
- Ask yourself if what you are worried about will really matter in five years. If the answer is no, then let it go. If yes, go back to that dark room to take a number of breaths.

Gain Perspective

- First, think about how lucky you are to be where you are. Find perspective by imagining that you're standing on a ladder where you can choose to look up or look down. Next, think about what you can do to feel better. Finally, do whatever you need to in order to distract yourself from the problem at hand.
- Think about others who have been through something similar and have somehow managed to live a full, happy life.
- Get clear about what is really bothering you. Stress causes the mind to swirl, so at first, you may feel there are too many problems to tackle. If you stop and list them, you're likely to find that what is swirling in your mind are the same two or three things, or variations of them. Once you pinpoint a manageable number of issues, you'll feel empowered to be able to manage them.
- Tell yourself that the situation you find yourself in will transition to something else and, ideally, something better. People in stress tend to believe that their current

feeling will never go away. Visualize a trolley ride in San Francisco, hang on for dear life through all of the bumps, and you will eventually get to the next stop.

- Understand and appreciate the life force. The frailty of the human condition gives rise to an unlimited number of possibilities and situations. Sometimes life happens in linear order, or as you planned or wanted, but most of the time, it's random. Issues overlap and intersect, one event may beget another, and you may have good and bad things happening to you all at the same time. You may look at others and think they are lucky but chances are, they have, or will go through, their own pain.

- If at night, you can't control the nagging thoughts, get out of bed and write down every unfinished piece of business that is tormenting you. Then assign times when you will deal with each problem.

- Think about how things could be worse and be thankful that they are not.

Find an Outlet

- Punch the crap out of a boxing bag three times a week for several months.

- Get a friend and set a workout routine or get a personal trainer.

- Do a Sudoku puzzle and let yourself feel proud when you complete it.

- Have a good cry and let it all out.

- Take a nice hot bath while sipping a glass of wine.
- Dance and listen to music to release tension.
- Move, whether that's dancing in the living room or taking a walk in nature, with music in your ears.
- Once a day, do something you really enjoy.
- Resume or re-establish exercise and consistently work toward a short-term goal to stay clearheaded.
- Get regular manicures. When you feel like your best, you feel more in control of yourself. On days when you feel terrible, dress really nicely. It is like you are dressing for success—or sometimes battle.
- Do something you love and be present. Listen to music, read, spend time with your kids, go for a hike.
- Find a television series to get addicted to or a great book to immerse yourself in.
- Exercise is a key stress reducer. A long run or ride can help you think through things. The healthier you are, the more equipped you are to handle stress and the happier you feel as a result.
- If you wake up feeling blue, as if you're facing a mountain, get active. The day will seem less daunting and you'll feel, well, happier. It's that simple.
- Read as many books as you can to immerse yourself in another world, with different problems that don't belong to you. Choose books that make you cry so you can let it out.

Seek Normalcy

- When life feels chaotic, maintain as normal a routine as possible. Go to work, coach hockey, don't give up your hobbies. You need some measure of control to keep the stress level under control.
- Make sure to go to bed at the same time every night and to wake up at the same time every morning. Doing so sets a stable routine, one that you desperately need in trying times.
- Make sure that everything is put away when you go to sleep at night. That way, in the morning, your house will feel under control.

LESSON 13

Live with No Regrets

Don't cry because it's over, smile because it happened.

– Dr. Seuss

We used to call our Grandfather "Bampa." He was a strong-minded man who always knew what he wanted from life. If he loved you, boy, did you know it. Every time I would ask him how he was doing, he had the same answer. He would look deep into my eyes and deliver the same line, "No regrets."

I believed him because his focus was always facing forward, not behind. As a result, any decision he made, he stood by. In the end, his choices might not always lead to the result he planned or hoped for, but so be it. The future was what mattered now, not the past. I loved his perspective and I learned from it.

Letting the past go, letting it rest where it is, sounds easy, but it's not. We are humans and, as such, we are going to stumble through life, making mistakes along the way. How do we live without regretting some of the choices that, in hindsight, were not the best ones?

Making decisions is a hard process for me. After much weighing of pros and cons, I try to settle on one side or the other and then it happens. I find myself in a constant state of second guessing. It doesn't make a difference whether the decision is big or small, I get obsessive. My brain wants to analyze every angle to avoid making a mistake or, even worse, failing.

Contemplation is not a bad thing and, in fact, it can be informative. It helps you to get clear about what you want and need, what your gut is telling you. But when analysis becomes paralyzing, that's when you know it's decision time already.

Is there a possibility that you can make the "wrong" decision? Is there a possibility that you'll live to regret it? That depends on your perspective, which is wholly within your control.

The fact is, no matter how hard we try to live without regret, we will trip up. Each day is long and busy, and we make so many choices along the way. So I always end my day with a dedicated time of reflection. Late at night, when the lights are out and the house is silent, I lie in bed and ask myself three important questions that will help me avoid feelings of regret.

1. Was I good to myself today?
2. Was I good to others?
3. Did I do the best that I could?

Most nights, I tick off each question with a resounding yes and go to sleep. But not always. Sometimes, I realize that I may have said something that I shouldn't have said. I may have deprived myself from taking care of my basic needs. I may have failed to give it my best shot. When the answer is no, what happens? It means I need to do some reflecting, and decide how I want to go about addressing my actions or behaving differently in the future.

The best thing about asking myself these three questions is that it helps to wipe the slate clean for today. It allows me to start fresh tomorrow with a new chance to get the answers right.

How can you make sure that your decisions don't lead you down the torturous path of regret after they're made? I have learned that if I follow my gut instead of letting my brain take over, regret rarely follows. The brain is a powerful force and often we let it think so much that it takes over. Our brains analyze every angle, creating so much noise that we can't hear our hearts. And that's where we should be focusing our attention, a little further south.

I have learned that if you live with a full heart, you live a fulfilled life. Therefore, if you make decisions with your heart, you will feel fulfilled, regardless of the outcome. Rarely do I feel regret when I make open-hearted choices.

The one regret that I find plagues me more than any other is holding back from doing something I really want to do. While decisions can be scary because they can lead to failure, they are, at the very least, a sign of action. Even if you try and fail, at least you know you tried, and just that knowledge alone can be enough to keep you safe from regret. By failing to try, there are more un-answered questions that can lead to regret. What if I had tried? What would have happened?

Jacob taught me so much about life that by the time I turned 40, I knew I wanted to change direction. My heart was telling me to find a way to spread the messages I had learned. So I listened. I left my secure classroom of 24 students and hit the road, on a mission to develop the Project Give Back curriculum that I had built in my own classroom.

Without a bi-weekly paycheck, I basically took a year off, but worked harder than I had ever imagined working in my lifetime. I wanted to make sure that the curriculum was flexible enough to reach every person in every type of environment, and that took patient research. It meant I was teaching in 16 classes per week for free, tweaking the curriculum each and every time, making notes and changes, and then crossing them all out and making more notes and more changes, again and again and again. Each night, when the house was quiet, I would stay up until all hours, on a mission to get my project on track.

Some weeks, I remember writing more than 36 reports and calling 36 students to coach them on their upcoming presentations. I was exhausted—physically, mentally, spiritually. But I knew this: I needed to take this chance to make a dream come true or there would always be the regret that comes with failing to try.

Over the years, there have, of course, been some results we didn't like, that in retrospect, we could have avoided. Do I regret these "failures?" No, because they were necessary. They taught me what not to do going forward and that's valuable information.

When I think of having no regrets, I am reminded of a sermon I once heard entitled "Live Life the Way You Would Like to Be Eulogized." Morbid? Maybe. But imagine if we all lived life this way, continuously aware of the way we act, behave, treat others and ourselves.

While none of us is beyond reproach, I often think about whether in my daily life, I am behaving like my best self. If I were to leave this world tomorrow, would I have made an impact? How would I be remembered? Would I have left the right clues on the trail for my children to follow? Would they always hear my voice inside their heads and would the messages guide them through their greatest challenges and accomplishments?

The words of wisdom in that 20-minute speech changed the way I live. I especially love this line about the impact you have in life: Even when you think no one is watching, the camera is always rolling. Remember that when you act. People are always watching, especially your children.

Let's all consciously try to live the way we would like to be remembered. Life may seem short, but eternity lasts forever. If we live this way, how can we have any regrets?

To learn to live life without regrets, try implementing some of these suggestions into your days.

- Don't procrastinate by rethinking details over and over. If your brain is doing somersaults around a decision, find a quiet spot so you can hear your heart. When there is something you feel you must do, that's a good sign that you should go for it.
- Don't harp on the past. The past is gone and can't be changed. The present is where work needs to be done.

Use the past to your advantage by learning from it and moving forward, armed with more knowledge.

- Don't make the mistake of failing to do something you really want to do. There is inherent regret in being scared to try. Tell yourself it's better to "fail" than to fail to try.

- Live the way you want others to see you, how you want to be remembered.

- Emulate someone you admire. Ask questions and learn from the masters.

- Give yourself time each night to contemplate whether you made decisions you're happy with. Don't beat yourself up if the answer is no. Use that answer to wipe your slate clean and make changes tomorrow.

- Remember that mistakes can be addressed. Don't be afraid to apologize if you said something you later deem wrong or if you think you offended someone. We all make mistakes but not taking responsibility for those errors may lead to regret.

- Let people know how much you care about them. You don't always have to say it, but make sure that by your actions they know and understand how you feel.

- It's okay to take a do-over. If you are thinking, I should've, would've, could've, that's okay. You can always go back and try again.

LESSON 14

Smile – Even When You Don't Want To

I'm just happy to be here!

– Joe Goodbaum

Not too long ago, a close friend of ours passed away. Joey Good-baum was a family man and a community and business leader who left his mark on all who were lucky enough to know him. At Telus, the place where he hung his hat every day, he was loved, respected and admired.

If Joey Goodbaum had a motto in life, it was this: "I'm just happy to be here." Any time you asked Joe how he was feeling, he answered the same way because no matter how he felt, his happiness to be alive was more important. Joey always had a smile on his face and a kind word to say. At 56, he was diagnosed with pancreatic cancer and passed away just 2 months later. As he fought to live, with his family at his side throughout his battle, he just kept on repeating those words that came to define him: I'm just happy to be here!

If Jake could speak, he would echo Joey's sentiment. We all suffer through trying times in life. They are part of the journey. And yet, some of us seem to be able to muster a smile, even in the face of darkness.

If Joey could smile, if Jake can smile, why can't the rest of us? Look around—on the bus, at pedestrians, at drivers. Are people smiling, enjoying their day, enjoying their lives?

Every day, we wake up with a mental list of what needs to get done. As we move through the day, it feels like we are all in a rush to get to where we are going. We forget to enjoy the ride. And how long does it take to smile? Less than one second. It happens in a flash.

Try an experiment. Spend one day with a smile on your face, even if you don't feel like it, even if you feel that there's nothing to smile about. Then watch what happens around you.

No one feels like smiling all the time, not even me. Sometimes I fight it because I am too tired, or just don't feel happy at a particular moment. But when I force myself to smile, some kind of magic happens. I start to believe in the power of my smile and pretty soon, despite myself, my mood lifts. The best thing about smiling is that it's contagious. It gets mirrored back. And soon, your forced effort becomes a natural habit. The more you smile, the better you feel and others reflect that positive energy. You've started a trend.

Every time Jacob smiles, he inspires someone else to reciprocate the emotion, and he doesn't even know he's doing it.

Mark Stibich, a health aging expert, puts it this way, "Smiling can trick the body into helping you elevate your mood because the physical act of smiling actually activates neural messaging in your brain. A simple smile can trigger the release of neural communication boosting neuropeptides as well as mood-boosting neurotransmitters like dopamine and serotonin. Think of smiling like a natural anti-depressant." He goes on to add, "Studies have shown that smiling releases endorphins, natural pain killers, and serotonin. Together these three neurotransmitters make us feel good from head to toe. Not only do these natural chemicals elevate your mood, but they also relax your body and reduce physical pain. Smiling is a natural drug."

Is this just a common case of fake it until you make it? Actually, I believe it just might be.

We all feel better when we look our best. It gives us that boost of confidence we need to hold our heads a little higher and stand a little straighter. When we add a smile to that mix, somehow a sense of happiness is transferred from our lips to our brains and it is obvious to everyone. So why not smile whether you feel like it or not? It's good for our well-being, makes us look better, lifts our spirits and helps others to smile, too.

Happiness oozes out of young kids. I love watching them in the halls at school. Most children don't walk in a straight line, putting one foot after the other. Instead, they skip, they hop, they jump to get to where they're going. These happy movements illustrate what's going on inside their young bodies. Every time I see a child skipping along the halls, I look at their face and there it is, a sweet smile.

So I tried it, just to see how I felt. I was on a walk, and I found myself alone on a street, no cars or people in sight. I looked to the left and the right, saw no one around, so I did it. I skipped. Just like those kids in the hallways. Instantly, I felt an inner sense of innocence and joy. (I bet you are smiling too, just imagining it.) Even though no one was there to see me, I couldn't help but giggle to myself. Skipping felt great and I felt so silly, but so empowered. I loved every second of it. I was smiling from the inside out, and I wanted to share that feeling.

That day, I went straight home and dared my children to try to skip without smiling. Both Bev and Ben were in. They took me up on the challenge and failed miserably. They couldn't do it. In just seconds, they were skipping but not as hard as they were laughing. That childhood joy had taken over and, like me, they couldn't resist it. And neither could my girlfriends, who were next on my skip challenge hit list.

We all want to feel happy and joyful, to recapture the delight of our youth but somewhere along the way, outside influences—adult ones—hinder us from skipping along. We have to find that beat and learn how to grab hold of our own childlike innocence, regardless of age.

Jacob's illness, although devastating at times, has managed to protect him from losing his childhood joy. Just being near him allows me to feel that skip in my step. It gives me strength to take that walk around in the world with energy inside me. If Jake can smile, then so can I.

So how do we do it? How do we manage to put a smile on our face when it may be the last thing we want to do? Here are some strategies to help you find your smile when you need it most.

- As soon as you wake up in the morning, think of three things that make you happy. Start your day with a smile and it will keep finding a way to reappear.
- Find a time when you are alone and skip. Start with just a couple of skips and take note of what happens inside your body. Dare your loved ones to take the skip challenge, too.
- When you're around other people, put a smile on your face. Then count how many smiles you see mirrored back.
- Put on some happy music, even for a minute or two, and crank it up. Better yet, belt out your favorites while in the shower or when driving your car.
- Call someone who makes you feel good inside—just to say hi. Tell them you just called to hear their voice. You can literally hear a smile in a voice from the other end of the phone. Relish in it, remember it, use it when you need a smile.

LESSON 15

The Marriage Equation – Give 90%; Take 10%

Real giving is when we give to our spouses what's important to them whether we understand it, like it, agree with it, or not.
— Michele Weiner Davis

Like most couples, when Jeff and I were married, we traded vows we believed would endure throughout our lives together. More than 20 years ago, we both spoke these ancient Hebrew words, "Ani l'dodi, ve dodi li," which mean "I am my beloved's and my beloved is mine." When the promise crossed our lips, we were so young, so in love and we couldn't wait to begin our lives together. Sharing our strong and promising vow would be the foundation for a marriage based on loyalty, trust, support and a lifetime of sharing. (As long as he didn't force me to share my french fries and popcorn, we'd survive. Some things are just not meant to be shared.) We were in it together, for the long run. I had his back and he had mine.

We were living a fairy tale but even in fairy tales, there are challenges to overcome. Like most successful marriages, ours has presented serious challenges and, yet, it has emerged as our biggest triumph, as we are always in it together.

Relationships are work, hard work, the hardest work that exists. They are composed of two very different individuals living together in (relative) harmony with their own unique predispositions. And so, it's no wonder that when life gets messy, we tend to regress. In fact, the harder things get, the quicker each of us regresses to what Jeff calls our three-year-old selves. Now, we've got two toddlers, who were born into two very different families with contrasting viewpoints and values, trying to solve problems together. It's not an easy task.

Here's the loop my husband and I kept finding ourselves in. As adults behaving like toddlers, we would get stuck. Unable to find common ground fast, we'd both retreat to our corners, except that retreat would look different for each of us. I'd break down in tears while Jeff would get angry. At the beginning of our relationship, we agreed that we would never go to bed angry. Not so easy when you're divided.

Over the years, we have gained a lot of wisdom about dealing with conflict in marriage. For starters, we have learned that time apart can calm us both down. Space often leads us back to each other and to a productive resolution, especially when tempers are exploding. What we realized is that our three-year-old selves both desperately need a time out before we can see eye to eye.

When life is good, marriage feels like it's the glue holding love strong. When life is challenged, though, that's when marriage is put to its test. Whether the obstacle is a difference in core values, illness or financial struggles, sometimes it seems as if our marriages are constantly on trial.

We are often asked how our marriage has managed to survive through caring for a chronically ill child 24/7. It's a sobering question. The fact is, recent research shows that when parents care for a child with special needs, divorce rates increase from 50 percent to more than 80 percent and it's no wonder.

After Jacob was diagnosed with Canavan Disease, Jeff and I went our separate ways, emotionally at least. In order to cope, we had no choice but to distance ourselves from each other. He crawled inside himself to deal with his grief the best way he knew how. For my part, I needed to get it all out, to talk, cry and share. We were divided, both soothing ourselves alone.

When we finally sought professional help, we found solace in the therapist's analogy. "I can see why you two are having such difficulty," she said. "In your marriage, you've got Marcia Brady and the Lone Ranger. How is that supposed to work?"

After a lot of thought, we figured it out. The only way our marriage could work was if Jeff allowed Marcia to be Marcia and I allowed the Lone Ranger be the Lone Ranger. We were never going to see things in the same way, from the same vantage point. We would never have the same personality or coping mechanisms. In order for us to be in sync with one another going forward, we had to accept each other for who we are.

Our therapist asked us to draw up a list of all the things that we needed from one another. Our answers taught us so much. My list was all about getting more attention from him, acts of kindness and togetherness. Jeff's was based on alone time and independence. Since that time, whenever we feel we are on rocky ground, no matter the situation or the challenge, I review our lists to remind myself of what we both need.

Through this process, the crux of our conflict has become clear, and it's never the problem we think it is. Instead, what's stalemating us is neglecting each other's needs. Although sometimes we forget, we always come back to the fact that Jeff can't be Ellen and Ellen can't be Jeff. For us to be a strong force in our union, we have to give up trying to change one another into ourselves and accept who we each are and who we are not.

Over the past two decades, our mutual acceptance has reaped many rewards. One is that we have allowed ourselves to learn from each other and as a result, we have both changed for the better. Living with a strong, independent man, I have become stronger and more independent. Being around a warm woman, Jeff has become warmer. Without even realizing it, we have subliminally given each other the gift of our own strengths just by giving in to the other person's needs. As we learned to respect and admire each another's differences, we become more similar, and our marriage grows stronger.

But as in any relationship, the work never ends. Although our marriage may be stronger than ever, we can never take each other for granted. As soon as we do, there is that old conflict again.

At our wedding, our Rabbi gave us a gift, the key to a successful marriage. He said, "The only way your marriage is going to work is if you both give 90% and only take 10%." The prophecy turned out to be true. When I give Jeff what he needs, he feels content as part of a partnership and our relationship thrives. Similarly, when he fulfills my needs, I am strengthened by his love for me and I love him even more. When we both give much more than we take, we are a team.

In a poll of couples who have been successfully married for more than 50 years, I asked both partners to share the special sauce in their recipe for a strong marriage. Here are their answers.

- Be an active listener.
- Resist fighting when you are angry. Wait until the steam settles.
- Pick each other up rather than pulling each other down.
- Space is just as important as togetherness.
- Give little unexpected surprises, such as bringing home flowers for no reason or calling to say, "I got dinner tonight, don't worry about it."
- Do something that you know your spouse does not like to do—fill the car with gas, take out the garbage, shovel the driveway.
- God gave us two ears and one mouth for a reason: Always listen before you speak.
- Treat one another with great respect. Children learn from what they see and not from what you tell them.

- Believe strongly in God and ask, on a daily basis, for his help and guidance.
- Enjoy doing certain activities together, but give each other enough space to do your own thing.
- True love is putting the other person first and knowing that it's okay to give in and you don't have to always be right.
- Always look out for your partner until eventually it becomes a habit.
- Know your partner's strengths and trust those strengths.
- Always take time for meaningful tenderness.
- Always have laughter in your lives and don't take yourself too seriously.
- When Mother respects Father and Father respects Mother, this trickles down to children respecting everyone.
- Make each other giggle. When you get older like us, it becomes even more important.

The Bonding Power of Siblings

The other night I ate at a real nice family restaurant.
Every table had an argument going.

– George Carlin

Siblings ground us with their honesty. They are our peers, our foils and our partners in crime. They are always there whether you like it or not.

Siblings call out every shot, so we can't get away with anything. They have a way of putting us in our place like no one else can. They know just the right button to press to get under our skin and they know the exact way to comfort us in our times of deep sadness or stress. They teach us how to share and how to be selfish, too, in the natural competition for parental attention. Our brothers and sisters are our people. Having known us forever, they will "get us" wherever our lives turn out. They will relate to the journey.

I have always been grateful for my two siblings. As a girl sandwiched between brothers, I feel like I am the youngest because

I have always looked up to each of them. The fact that they are both over 6-foot-3 helps fuel that dynamic. Like all sibs, though, we had our moments, ones that ended with slamming doors or screaming lungs. A ping pong racquet thrown at my head or a hidden shove when our parents weren't looking was standard stuff. But let's face it, siblings keep us humble and strengthen our character. One thing I have always known in my gut is that, without a doubt, these guys have my back and I have theirs.

As a young girl, I remember watching how my friends interacted with their brothers and sisters. It often seemed like a war zone, a minefield, where fights can erupt out of almost nowhere. Sound familiar?

Now that I have my own three children, the sibling interaction is back. But watching Bev and Ben grow up as Jacob's younger siblings is an extraordinary sight to witness. They have a bond that goes beyond the typical brother-sister relationship. For good or bad, they have a different experience.

When our kids were young, we couldn't just pick up and go out as a family. Everything took great planning, effort and time. Jake's siblings had to get used to continuously waiting for their older brother to get ready. They had to insert themselves into that process. They had to help out. The patience and helpfulness that Bev and Ben learned growing up became part of who they are. Today, they are first to open doors, clear obstacles out the way, wipe off the car and run back in the house for anything that might have been forgotten. Helping out is in their blood.

When Bev and Ben are around Jake, they are especially tuned in to what he needs. They take turns in the back seat of the minivan sitting beside him so that when he coughs, they can offer help. They are the ones to push his head up and forward so he won't choke on his saliva. When they are kicking back watching a favorite show on TV, they have to tune out their brother's heavy breathing beside them. They are sympathetic and considerate toward us when they know we have had a rough night with Jake.

When either Bev or Ben is sad or frustrated, I have heard them sneak into each other's rooms to comfort one another. There is no better sound than the giggles we hear coming from behind a closed door.

Having a brother with such severe disabilities has impacted both Bev and Ben's lives in so many ways. But we didn't want Jake's life to be the defining force for them. We wanted both Bev and Ben to find their own unique passions that act as both an outlet and a hobby. We wanted them each to have something personal to grasp, especially when times get tough.

From a young age, both Bevvy and Ben tested out various activities to see which ones they enjoyed. They tried so many of them: Soccer, baseball, football, dance, hockey and swimming. Bev was a fish in the swimming pool and Ben grabbed hold of that hockey stick and never let go. These outlets help to keep them active, driven and busy with their own lives.

Despite the fact that Jacob is very different from them in so many ways, Bev and Ben adore their brother, and they are constantly learning from him. In Bev's grade 11 English class, she wrote a speech about the lessons she has learned from her older brother.

> I would like everyone to take a moment to think about your most treasured memory. One moment where you felt utter bliss. Maybe it was watching the sunset on the last night of summer. Or when you took the first bite of that really good burger. Maybe it was the feeling when you finished that race for which you've trained for months. Now imagine if you couldn't see that sunset. Couldn't swallow that burger. And it would be impossible for you to ever finish that race. Right now you are imagining the life of my brother Jacob.
>
> Jacob was diagnosed with a rare disease called Canavan Disease that disrupts the way your brain sends messages though the body. Because of this, he will never be able to see, walk, eat or talk. And yet, Jacob is the happiest person I know.
>
> But how is this possible? How is it that someone who physically cannot see the world can have so much insight about what's going on around him? People who have had a greater struggle in life, like Jacob, end up having a better understanding of happiness because of their ability to remain positive, to appreciate even the smallest things, and because of the way they inspire others.

"Behind every exquisite thing that existed, there was something tragic," said Oscar Wilde in *The Picture of Dorian Gray.*

In order to be truly happy, appreciation is essential. It is hard to genuinely appreciate what surrounds you if you haven't experienced life without it. Never have I seen someone's face light up so brightly as Jacob's does from something as little as our father saying hello. Jacob appreciates his ability to hear because he's never had the need to see our father's expression to know that he is there.

Jacob has the ability to not only appreciate the things around him but the people around him. He understands that he wouldn't be able to survive without our parents and caregivers. He knows this from the constant care he needs. Physically capable teenagers in 2016 do not need that constant care so what your parents have done for you is more masked. Also, our own expectations play a huge part in our ability to appreciate. We tend to have high expectations of the people around us. For example, if our favorite artist doesn't perform well, we end up disappointed. Jacob has no expectations of anyone and because of that, he is satisfied by the little things in life.

There is one characteristic that can change a person's perspective on everything: Positivity. One thing that affects our positivity is the social media that surrounds us. You can't walk into a mall or down the street without seeing an ad that wipes out your self-confidence and then that same ad tells you how to fix yourself by buying their product. Jacob isn't exposed to this negativity and is therefore confident just as he is. The people that we choose to surround ourselves with also have a tremendous effect on how we behave. If we are constantly with people who tear themselves down, we will end up catching their negativity like a cold.

Jacob is a prime example of the opposite experience. If someone negative is around him, they can't help but end up smiling. Eventually, the person realizes that if someone who has such a severe illness can be happy, why can't they? Jacob can always find that silver lining.

Jacob has made so many of us better people. He has shown everyone around him how to live. To not take one day for granted. One of the worst feelings is regret and if you live each day to its fullest, you will rarely have regret. He also teaches us the meaning of empathy. The ability to see a situation from a different perspective can change your actions for the better. If you give back, live life to its fullest and become empathetic, you will be able to achieve a greater happiness.

In this day and age, when we have so much, we tend to take life for granted. We never take a step back to realize how lucky we really are to be able to see, walk, eat and talk. Jacob cannot walk or see yet he has shown so many people the right way to live. My brother has turned me into the person I am today and I don't know where I would be without him teaching me how to try to stay positive as I appreciate the world around me.

As parents, there is no greater feeling than when we realize that our children are growing up to be strong, independent, caring and loving people.

We can only do our best and try to model what we feel is best for our own children. Jacob may not be the typical older brother— the guy who gives advice, protects them from harm or tests them to their limits. Instead, he has given his siblings other values. He has been a role model of human kindness, strength and resilience and for that, I am forever grateful.

Our siblings teach much more than we could learn in school. When I asked some friends what are the greatest lessons that they learned from their siblings, the answers were fascinating.

- We all turned out to be different, but when it comes right down to it, our values are the same. That gives me comfort.
- We just get one another.
- No matter what is going on, they will drop everything when I need them. No explanation needed.
- We share memories that make the word "forever" have true meaning.

- Whether a word, a place, a song or a name—common memories will always be with us.
- Growing up as the youngest of three girls, I learned from my sisters all about worldliness, confidence and how to ruin their appetites so I could have the last piece of cake.
- My sister is my angel, always keeping an eye out on me and for me. She has my best interests at heart. She understands and accepts me for who I am and loves me for it. I would do anything for her, anytime. We are fiercely protective of each other. She's taught me so much by example. I've always looked up to her. When we were young, I admired her athletic abilities and now I love her kind and fun nature. I hope that my bond with my sister inspires my kids to remain as close with their brothers as they get older.
- The older I get the more I learn how similar we are, which allows for healthy reflection.
- They make me giggle without trying—just one look, that's all it takes.
- No sugar coating, they say it as it is. That is something so rare, necessary and authentic.
- We look at one another and can tell what the other is thinking without saying a word.
- I don't need to try to be anyone else but me around my siblings.

Become Part of a Whole

One good thing about music, when it hits you, you feel no pain.

– Bob Marley

Jacob feels music. Without the ability to communicate through language, eye contact or physical gestures, music is his language. He speaks and understands it fluently. How do I know? As soon as Jake hears three strums on a guitar, his body signals understanding. His eyes widen, his mouth opens and there's that smile again. All we have to do is look at his eyes and we can see the life inside of him, dancing to the magic and power of music.

When Jacob turned 18, we knew we had hit a major milestone. It was one we hoped for but never expected to reach, and one that deserved a special celebration. We wanted to share our miracle with anyone who wanted to be part of it. We had a purpose and we definitely had a reason to celebrate. It was time to plan Jake's Jam: 18 songs representing 18 lessons symbolizing 18 years.

Just like Jake does, I wanted every person who participated in the concert, everyone in the room that night, to feel the music. Through Jacob's Ladder, we had built a tight-knit communal family, a unit that ended up so much larger than any of us could have imagined. Together, we managed to create an experience that had taken on a life and meaning of its own.

The first step was to reach out to our network of angels. I called everyone who had been part of the Jacob's Ladder family to tell them our next project and ask if they wanted to help. We started with our sponsors from past events. After I explained our vision, and expressed our hope for a presenting sponsorship in the amount of $18,000, the answer that came back was astonishing: But we were hoping for $25,000. And that was just the start. Every sponsor, every person, every company offered more than we could ever have asked for. They were all in, in, in, with everything they had to give.

Everyone knew that on April 30, 2015, there was going to be one sensational party not only celebrating Jacob's life, but celebrating the miracle of so many people who wanted to be part of it.

This time, our volunteers were sworn to secrecy about the details of Jake's Jam. We wanted everyone who attended to have Jake's experience, to be surprised and delighted by the feeling of music as it hit their souls. So we kept it all hush-hush from everyone—except Jacob, of course. He was in on every detail.

Jacob was our barometer. Any performer whose music he loved was invited to play. We didn't hold ordinary auditions. Some artists came to our house to sing for Jacob in person and some sang to him over the phone. It was easy to tell if it was a thumbs up. One shiny smile, and we knew they were in. Whether a musician was famous to the masses, or famous to us or not even necessarily famous, it didn't matter. If they shone in Jacob's eyes, they were sure to shine on the big stage.

Jackie Richardson was one of our performers. I had the pleasure of witnessing this award-winning gospel and blues singer in action at another charity event, months before Jake's Jam. Every note that comes out of Jackie's mouth is like a warm hug. There was no doubt that Jake would go mad for her gospel and bluesy tone. But contacting a star is not as easy as it sounds. So I went to work.

I called everyone I knew in the entertainment world, hoping for an in. I cold - called her, on the off-chance that she would answer. I dug up her e-mail address and sent a note. I Facebook friended her. I tried her on LinkedIn and Instagram. I even tracked down one of her agents. Finally, after exhausting every avenue I could think of, I discovered that one of my relatives knew her and, just like that, we were connected. After several e-mails back and forth, we set up a call.

Even her "hello" was all rhythm and pizzazz. I got right down to business. I told Jackie about Jake and the concert we were planning to celebrate his birthday. She let out this deep belly laugh that echoed across the line. I asked if I could put her on the speaker so Jake could meet her, too, and then her throaty voice soothed into the room: "Hi Jakey, I've been waiting to speak to you."

Jake's face lit up as he felt Jackie's energy in the room. She asked which song Jake would like to hear and I told her to choose. There was silence for a moment and then came her voice.

He's got the whole world in his hands, he's got the
whole wide world in his hands, he's got the whole world
in his hands, he's got the whole world in his hands.

It was clear from Jake's expression that he was hooked on the
sound, on the words, so I grabbed my cell phone and filmed the
connection. Before the call ended, I pushed the send button and
told Jackie to check her e-mail.

And there it was, right in front of her. When Jackie saw the
impact she had on my child just by singing four lines to a song,
the deal was sealed.

Finally, the highly anticipated evening arrived. The house lights
in the packed and sold-out Mirvish Panasonic Theatre in downtown Toronto went dark. All eyes focused onto the large screen at
the front of the theater. Jake's Uncle Rob created a video that set
the mood for the entire evening. We could all relate to the magical
power of music. He had captured this universal language that Jakey
speaks fluently and shared it with the entire audience. Without one
word spoken, we could all hear Jacob as we witnessed this love on
the massive screen in front of us.

Jackie Richardson opened the show with *He's Got the Whole
World in His Hands*. Jake was waiting behind the stage, drinking in
every note.

After Jackie drew in the audience with her soulful radiance, Jen
and Stacy sang directly to Jake, just as they do every Sunday afternoon. This time, though, there were 700 people in the completely

sold-out venue. We all felt as if we were at home, jamming in the Schwartz family room.

After Jen and Stacy's two sons joined us onstage to serenade Jake, out came four up-and-coming stars to perform. The audience could not believe the power that came out of their young voices. The talent continued with an award-winning show choir from the Etobicoke School of the Arts, composed of 50 teens, who danced, tapped and sang.

The audience was moved in every way—emotionally, spiritually, even physically. In our seats, we couldn't help but sway and dance. We surrendered to the wave of music and love. We were captivated by the amazing talent in front of us. It was a joyous ride. We were taken from our family room jam to the likes of Broadway and then to a campfire moment when four moms came together in perfect harmony to sing a folk song. They were followed by the director of a camp for children with special needs who led us in a communal singsong of the classic *Hallelujah*, together with three young teenage performers.

The next performer was Lil JaXe, a 16-year-old boy, who came out wearing khakis and a black t-shirt. With great effort, he began to speak. Lil JaXe told us how happy he was to be at Jake's Jam but it took some time for us to hear him. Lil JaXe has such a severe stutter that each syllable struggles to make its way out of him. Very slowly and with deliberation, he told his story and, as we sat there, uncomfortably captivated with bated breath, we hung on every word.

"Because of my stutter, I was picked on by kids and teachers. It has been like that for all of my life. Rap has saved me. It is an honor to be here performing for Jake's birthday. Happy Birthday, dude."

Lil JaXe said "Let's go," and to our surprise, when the boy began to sing, the stutter vanished. As if on cue, the audience lifted hands in the air and we swung our arms side to side to the beat of Lil JaXe's inspirational rap, an original song called *A Kid with a Dream*.

Next, our host of the evening, Mark Breslin, introduced Dana Rocket, owner of a spin studio in downtown Toronto. We all jumped out of our seats and shouted out the words along with her as she belted out the song *Carry On* by the American indie band Fun. "Whatever happens, whatever challenges we face we must carry on," sang Dana as we all danced together in place.

After intermission, the lights dimmed and there on the stage sat Bev and Ben. For weeks they had been working hard with two close friends to create an original song as a tribute to their brother. Accompanied by a good friend Don, they sang these words for the first time.

> Every morning his smile,
> It makes our day.
> His smile never fails to blow us away.
> Because of Jake we've learned to appreciate
> The difference a smile can make.
> Returning from school, walking through the snow
> We see Melda bouncing Jake to the radio.

> Because of Jake we've learned the power of music to
> inspire.
> Jake's courage and spirit inspire us to always reach
> higher.
> We know cuz we've spent our whole lives learning from
> Jacob.
> We know, cuz we've found the best of ourselves,
> Because of him.

As if our hearts weren't touched enough, Hayden Desser, known only as Hayden, took the microphone and shared this story. "I wrote this song for my daughter. She is five years old and she has special needs. She is non-verbal, but like Jake, she loves music. I wrote this song in her honor. It's called *No Happy Birthday*."

As he sang this tribute to honor his child, the audience leaned in, hoping along with him, "Maybe one day you'll sing along."

Next, Kenny Munshaw serenaded the crowd with his warm and welcoming music and Amy Sky sang her hits, *I Will Take Care of You* and *Ordinary Miracles*.

There was one more surprise. A famous celebrity gave a live feed personal serenade straight from his Los Angeles living room. The song was projected onto a huge screen that transported us all into another place and time. Who was it? I'll never tell. Some things that happen at Jake's Jam remain at Jake's Jam.

It was yet another celebration we would carry with us forever. As usual, the event was composed solely of donations—everything from the venue, the directors, the gifts, the lighting, the sound, the printing costs, the delicious food and the spectacular talent. Music was at the heart of the gala and, like a symphony orchestra, everyone involved contributed to the feeling. We all felt lucky to be there, in the vulnerability that comes when you let yourself feel love in a room. Perfect harmony was created not only by the music, but by the hundreds of people who gathered together to unite in love. Every detail was planned and orchestrated with love, about love and for love, but there was no way to create that feeling. It was conjured by the people who were in the room, who gave of themselves in the most charitable way.

The energy at Jake's Jam was electric. Every bottom in every seat felt invested and honored to be at this celebration. Every person, every company wanted to be a part of the larger whole. Everyone contributed without a fee or hesitation.

When I tried to thank every supporter, the answer kept coming back the same, "You helped me more than I was able to help you."

Looking back at Jake's Jam, I am always amazed by all of the people and companies who gave all they could for a cause they support. We watch, we learn, we take it all in and I am forever grateful.

How can you become part of a cause and feel that connection to the greater good? Start by looking around you.

- The first step is easy. Just pick up the phone and ask how you can help.
- What is your talent? Find a charity that you care about and lend that talent out. We have a friend named Lisa

who is a visionary in marketing and design. Seventeen years ago, she offered her services and she has contributed ever since.

- Most charities are dependent on any help they can get. Time is one of the most valuable gifts you can give. If you have some time on your hands, offer it to the charity of your choice.

- There is no job beneath you when volunteering for a charity. When you offer to help, be committed and ready to do anything. We have a few volunteers who pack up after every event. These energetic people are invaluable because they take over in moments of exhaustion.

- Be prepared to meet like-minded individuals who care and want to help just like you. Nothing is more fulfilling than the connection of charitable souls.

Life Goes On, Whether We Like It or Not!

Yesterday is history. Tomorrow is a mystery.
Today is a gift. That's why it is called the present.

– Alice Morse Earle

The other day, I looked over at Jacob and was shocked by what I saw. His eyes rolled back in their sockets, his head jerked to the right and his breathing seemed to stop.

"Jake, Jake?"

No response.

His body was frozen except for his right thumb rhythmically thumping up and down matched by the right side of his upper lip quivering to that same beat.

I went into mother mode. While rubbing his shoulders, I kept assuring him, over and over, "It's okay, Jakey. You are going to be okay." How did I know that? Why was I saying that? I had no clue whether or not he was going to be okay. But that's what we do as parents; we try to make everything better. To my relief, 30 seconds or so later, Jake's breath returned. Then his eyes rolled around and settled in the center position while the right side of his lower lip hung down. This was something we hadn't seen before. What was happening? Was it a seizure? Was it a stroke?

The doctor advised us to watch Jacob carefully. Over the course of the next few days, there were two more similar episodes, but thankfully, they were short-lived. We were getting used to the process of being vigilant.

We booked an EEG with Jake's neurologist. While the results didn't measure seizure activity, the doctor suspected one based on the symptoms. We went home with an increased dose of medication and the satisfaction that we had everything under control.

Then something drastically changed. Every few minutes, Jacob's head would move to the right and we knew what would follow. Soon, the seizures were coming on fast and furious, and we were documenting each one. Once we hit 50, we stopped counting, and back we went to the hospital for an MRI to find out what was happening inside Jacob's body. Most MRI patients are stressed out by this claustrophobic, loud and scary test. Jacob loved every beep, bump and sound. We did not love the results, however.

Jacob's disease had progressed. The images showed us what we had all feared: A severely diseased brain. Sadness and fear were threatening to engulf me. The worst could happen soon. The time that we were borrowing, that had been on loan for the last 19 years of Jacob's life, might be coming to an end.

Over the past few years, we have slowly watched Jacob's health deteriorating. The signs of decline were clear. There was a time when we didn't need to take the suction machine with us on outings. Now Jacob needed this life-saving vacuum by his side at all times. There was no way we could miss the fact that his breathing had become more labored as well.

Instead of harping on the sadness of Jacob's decline, we consciously trained our minds to enjoy every moment with him.

Now, though, we could no longer avoid the future. Suddenly, we were forced to look through the window into a world without Jacob, a world that we have avoided for almost two decades.

No matter what happens, this book is a testament to a life that, in its own small way, has changed not just me, but also anyone in Jake's world. In it are the valuable lessons that Jacob has taught me about how to appreciate every moment on Earth and how to bring meaning to each one. What better way to preach what you practice than to first practice what you preach?

Although the lessons in this book guide me all the time, I, like everyone, need constant reminders. When I am at my lowest, I will reflect on what each one has taught me, and conjure the feelings of comfort they bring. I will let them guide me through the difficult days that lay ahead. I hope that you will reach for them as well in your times of need.

We can't change the challenges we face but we can change how we deal with them. We will get through the toughest times but exactly how we survive is always up to us, day by day, step by step. Robert Frost wrote, "In three words I can sum up everything I've learned about life: It goes on." Let's make life go on in the best possible way, and let's do it together, with all the love and support we can muster.

We plan and God laughs. The best we can do is smile back and be thankful for the ride.

In the Raw,
by Jeff Schwartz

I'm not a writer, and when you consider that along with me being described as The Lone Ranger, you can imagine how challenging it is to write something open and authentic about our son Jacob. And yet, that is exactly what Ellen asked of me. Her intentions were good. She wanted a perspective on the lessons learned from our child from someone else with a similar relationship to him. The problem was, I was simply not up to the task.

Very early in our marriage, when things began to get stressful, a counselor described our union as "Marcia Brady Meets the Lone Ranger." While Ellen gained her strength from sharing, I gained mine from introspection. So it made sense that writing a chapter on my perspective of life with a disabled child, and what I learned from it, wasn't high on my bucket list, let alone something I felt comfortable doing. In fact, as I started to think about how I would approach this task, I wasn't even sure I could do it. For a long time, opening a "new blank document" in Word was about as I far as I could get. I even tried talking it out, by creating a few voice memos on my phone whenever an idea struck. But I was stuck.

Not one to give up on a challenge, I turned to my forum group members for help. I have been friends with these business colleagues for almost 20 years, and 8–10 times a year, for 4 hours at a time, we meet and talk. The cornerstone of this group is no judgment and, above all, everything spoken within it is confidential. The members know me, and I know them.

So when I brought my conundrum to the table, they were ready with guidance. The answer was clear. Ultimately, we all decided that I would never forgive myself if I didn't honor Ellen's request. But still the question remained: How? An idea came to me soon after. The group members would ask me questions and I would answer them. Writing my perspective might be hard, but surely, I could answer a few questions! So here is my take on the lessons learned from Jacob.

How much do you love your son?

I love him tons.

When he is gone, it will leave a huge void in my life. Why? Because of who I am, especially at my most vulnerable. Is this a character judgment of me? Yes. Is this a cop out, insomuch as I am not comfortable with sharing my feelings openly for fear of judgment or a response that doesn't make me comfortable with those feelings? Yes, this is a cop out. I am an introvert, taking the easier way of not sharing openly because I just want those feelings to be. Because I don't want a response, because I don't want something solved and because I just want to pour my feelings out at that moment. Jacob allows me and encourages me to do that with his smile and the hope that I will receive one. What will I do when he is gone?

What sacrifices have you made for him?

None. I have made no sacrifices for Jacob. I have helped to cater our lifestyle around his needs, but these are not sacrifices. He is my son. They are just his needs.

For Ben, I will get up early, I will drive carpool, I will sit around a hockey rink while he prepares for his next game. For Bevvy, I will get up early, so early that the first number on the clock is a four, and I will devote a weekend in a hot steamy pool to see her swim for a total of five minutes. These are not sacrifices. These are just things you do as a father, as a parent, because you want to, because you want to give your children every chance of success and participation in life.

Do I view this as being selfless? No. If the definition of selflessness, or sacrifice, means that you forego your own personal needs and desires for those of someone else, the answer is still no. I am getting tremendous satisfaction and joy (most times) from watching my kids participate, succeed and grow. It is the same with Jacob, just on a different level, with different expectations. With Jacob, my joy comes from getting that smile, when his face literally opens up with brightness. It comes from watching him sleep restfully and rhythmically, without wrestling for air. It comes from being there when he gets a great cough and freeing his body from the phlegm that is constricting and encumbering his breathing. And then, from the requisite deep breath and sigh that follows this accomplishment. What's better than that?

What has he taught you?

I don't know. I often get asked this question, and I really don't know. Isn't that the purpose of this book? Can I be so bold as to say that I have learned nothing? Maybe I have tapped into my feelings, my knowledge and my experience in a way that is not typical. If this is a question for comparison to what other people have learned in their lives, how can I say that mine is special or different in some way?

I wrestle with this question because maybe in some way, I feel that I am not "deep" enough to understand, appreciate or identify what these lessons are. And in some way, perhaps I am avoiding learning them because (I am crying as I am writing this; there is a nerve there somewhere) I feel deep down spiritually that I am supposed to learn lessons from Jacob and, if I do, part of his life's mission will be achieved and his work will be done. I am not ready to face that possibility. I would rather be shallow and dumb than lose him.

How has what Jacob has taught you impacted other parts of your life?

Now this question is dependent on the previous question; if I have not learned lessons, then how would they impact other parts of my life? Let's look at the question this way: What changes have I noticed in the way I live my life, the way I approach events and situations that I find myself in, and the way I treat people? I am not quite sure where the impact is manifesting itself, but I do believe I am a more spiritual person than I thought I would or could be. To me, being spiritual means that I pay more attention to my actions and my words. I evaluate whether how I am about to react to something will be a reflection of my personal values, something I am willing to be held accountable for. Accountable to whom? To my spouse, to my children, to my friends, to my extended family? Yes and no. Yes, because I care about how these people think about me to a certain degree. No, because I am accountable to a higher power. This is the point where the spirituality comes in, the point where I feel I have changed. Am I true to this type of evaluation 100 percent of the time? No, I am not. But there is no doubt that my needle has moved closer to the 100 percent mark than it was before life with Jacob.

For me, observance is the degree to which someone will follow the laws and rituals of one's faith. While I do not characterize myself as an observant person, I do believe I am a spiritual person and that there is a higher power that is looking over us and judging our behavior. As a result of this belief, I spend more time thinking about my values, what's important in my life and making sure that my actions reflect those values.

Here is a short story that took me somewhere I would not have gone many years ago. One weekend a group of eight of us were sitting outside having an enjoyable conversation. Quickly, the topic turned to a group of people who weren't with us and began examining their behaviors, not in a positive way. While I am no saint, talking about others in a negative way, especially if they are not present, makes me uncomfortable and turns me very quiet. This was not always the case. In the past, I would happily chime in without hesitation. But this time, I tuned out so much that I fell asleep, right there in the middle of the conversation. Now I often ask myself, if I am answerable for my actions to a higher power, wouldn't it have been the right thing to stand up for the people who were the subject of that conversation? How come I didn't step in and voice my opinion? Those are questions that I struggle with and I can point to specific situations where had I stepped in, it wouldn't have ended well. Who am I to judge other people's behavior just because it differs from mine?

Early on, when Jacob first left a stroller for a wheelchair and we would take walks in the neighborhood, we received mixed reactions. There were both stares and friendly greetings, and we learned to appreciate both. Then there were those conversations where others complained about how their lives had been turned upside down—as a result of the most minor issues. Ellen and I tried to rationalize their experiences but we couldn't. How could they be so upset? Really, are they kidding? Let them walk a day in our shoes; that will teach them.

Ultimately, we found ourselves feeling bitter and resentful about how people reacted to life's twists and turns. Sometimes, the lack of perspective even changed our opinion of close friends until one day, I said to Ellen, "If we keep this up, we won't be able to talk to anyone anymore. We won't have any friends and we'll resent everyone we know. We don't know what goes on when we're not around, so who are we to judge? There are very few in our particular situation, and we are by no means perfect. We handle things in our own way and many others may not agree with how we approach life. And that's okay." This change in attitude helped both of us to understand others, helped us to listen and to reflect on how we reacted to the events in our life. There are still times when I will comment if I feel the need, but it is only after much consideration and always meant to be constructive, not destructive.

What advice would you have for fathers of children with or without disabilities?

This is a tough question, and when I think about it, I should address it from two points of view. Why am I writing this chapter from the viewpoint of a father? Yes, I am Jacob's dad but these are just a parent's opinions and feelings. They could just as easily belong to a mother. The impact that Jacob has had on my life is not unique to me. He has had a similar impact on the lives of Ellen and our children, and anyone else who has been touched by him.

The second viewpoint applies to anyone with children who are special. Bring them into your lives in any and every way you can. That's a pretty sweeping statement, and that's not for everyone, but for me, it was clear from the beginning that wherever, whenever and however it was possible, we were going to include Jacob in our lives. Doing so has been so rewarding, but it hasn't been easy. Even the most ordinary activities, like going for a walk or out for dinner, take two-to-three times longer than it would in other families, but really, outings just take planning and time.

Having Jacob be a part of almost everything we do has not only enriched all of our lives but I truly believe it's one of the reasons that Jacob is still with us. Exposing, even immersing, Jacob in seemingly ordinary family outings and events stimulates him in ways we could not have dreamed possible when we first started this journey. In the process of including Jacob, we have developed bonds with people outside our family as well as rituals we count on. If throughout this journey, I had kept our family life and struggle private, we would have missed out on the family and community bonding that has been so enriching for Jacob and everyone who comes into contact with him.

One more short story on the topic of advice and inclusion. In a Jewish family, it is customary for a boy to have a Bar Mitzvah upon reaching the age of 13. In the years leading up to Jacob's 13th birthday, Ellen and I would sit down at quiet moments, usually early weekend mornings, and plan this milestone. We would literally visualize the entire event before taking step one in executing it. A nice, quiet, semi-private event on a Sunday (Bar Mitzvahs are traditionally on a Saturday morning) at the synagogue with extended family and that was it. We approached the Rabbi of our synagogue with our plan confident in our ideas and ready to go. However, this is where things began to change, rapidly and dramatically.

Our Rabbi had another approach, one that Ellen and I had not considered and was vastly different than our own. However it was his delivery that surprised us both. Initially, he agreed with our idea as a potential option and then he followed with the words, "However you will be robbing your community of something very special." Ouch, we hadn't considered that, or even contemplated that path as something the congregants would even consider. Ultimately, that was the route we chose and the whole experience was something that our friends and congregants of the synagogue still talk about some six years later. It truly was an uplifting experience for all who witnessed it. Without this type of inclusion and acceptance it would not have been possible.

How much do you love your wife and what does she mean to you?

In the book, Ellen provided her perspective on marriage, and I think she did a great job. In fact, I approved the content, and my approval is not a husband's autocratic last word. Rather, it's a symbol of the mutual respect we share. All marriages go through ebbs and flows, and ours is no different. Early on, after the "courting phase" and the first years of marriage, our relationship wasn't pretty. After some brief counseling, we found that we were trying to change each other into ourselves rather than enjoying what attracted us to each other in the first place.

This cycle caused friction between us that was exacerbated in stressful moments. Let me tell you, learning how to care for your first child who is disabled was the definition of stressful. It wasn't until Jacob became more stable and we learned to respect each other's point of view that our relationship started to improve. Of course, in times of stress, we still retreat to our two-year-old selves and there's that friction again, but it doesn't happen often. More importantly, our respect for each other is now so immense that we have become each other's loudest cheerleaders.

Ellen is a perpetual source of inspiration to me. It's almost as if, over the course of the last ten years, she has found her voice and now she is shouting from the rooftops. Hers is an amazing transformation to behold. In some small way, I have helped to create the opportunity for her to grow and I can't help but feel a little pride as a result. The downside, if there is one, is that I find it hard not to compare her growth to mine, and I am not yet at that point.

Last night, my daughter said something to me in jest, and after 22 years of marriage, it made my spirits soar. She said, "Dad, you guys are just like a young couple!" And you know, that's how I feel, young and in love.

What do you hope to achieve by writing this chapter?

I'm not sure. It began as a request from Ellen as a contribution to her book. The idea was that I might capture something from my viewpoint as a male and as a father of a disabled child that she cannot. As well, I imagine Ellen hoped that I might gain something from the experience of expressing myself, that it would be cathartic to get my feelings out there so that I may be able to understand and appreciate them even more (hmmm, is that Ellen trying to move me closer to her point of view?). The reality is that the exercise has been cathartic, wonderful and a nightmare—all at the same time. As I said to a friend, sometimes we have to leave our comfort zone and push ourselves to do things that are against our nature so that greatness can result.

If there is anything that I have learned in my years as Jacob's dad, as a father, as a husband and as an adult functioning in today's society, it is that my questions, my experiences and my attitudes are not unique. If I am experiencing a challenge, if I have questions, there is someone else out there who has encountered a similar situation with value to share. Just as I learn from those around me, I am hopeful that my words will resonate and benefit others in some small way.

What is your relationship like with your other two children?

Ellen and I wanted to give our two other children as normal an upbringing as we possibly could. That meant sports, interests, independence and guidance on an individual level, all of which can be achieved with planning.

By grade four, we had all agreed Bevvy's talents would not be in team sports, or any sport that required a ball. She naturally gravitated towards swimming and without any experience, she made her school swim team and did well in competition. At the end of the year, she came to me and asked if she could make swimming a "bigger part of her life." I said yes, of course, without knowing what I was getting myself into, without considering what life would be like as the dad of a swimmer.

I am no swimmer, having learned only enough to participate in other water sports. But almost a decade later, after learning to do the butterfly stroke, watching my daughter swim thousands of hours in the pool, recognizing that mornings start with a four as the first digit on a clock, eating twenty-five hundred calorie breakfasts and measuring time by the hundredth of a second, I am proud to say that Bevvy has developed one of her passions, and we helped her get there.

Ben, like me, developed more of an interest in team sports like hockey and all sports that required a ball. This was an easier transition as I was on familiar ground, maybe too familiar.

Whether it was Ben or Bevvy, for me, it was about being there, planning my schedule so that I could participate and share in their passions. Like many parents, Ellen and I became wizards at carpool and the divide-and-conquer method of parenting. This ideology has allowed me to coach many of Ben's teams throughout the years, and to bond with him through our common interests. If there is one sacrifice that both Ellen and I have made, it is that, depending on the circumstances, both of us can't be at all events at the same time.

It's amazing the bonding and growing that can take place when you incorporate time and interests in the same recipe. And yet, while we tried to provide the most "normal" upbringing for Bevvy and Ben, circumstances often intervened. Both of them are champs and I believe they have grown as a result of their experiences.

Ellen fondly remembers the time she spent with her father growing up, sharing common interests like tennis, travel and checking out the best steak houses and ice cream parlors. She encouraged me to do the same with our children. What she was really saying was that it was important for them to have time with their father doing "normal" fun things.

For the three of us, that meant primarily one thing: Waterskiing. This is one of those activities that falls under the divide-and-conquer category. While I have always been resistant to travel for extended periods because that means long periods of "on time" with Jacob, indulging this passion was important and we (mostly Ellen) would often make the necessary sacrifices. Today, if you ask either Bevvy or Ben to recount their most memorable experiences, they will talk about being on the water during the summer or taking waterski trips in the winter with their dad. Those memories are ones I cherish, too. To be able to put all the extra "time and planning" aside for a brief period and experience life like many fathers do has been a real treat.

As a father, I am fiercely dedicated to doing my share and making a contribution. There is really nothing special about that, I am sure that many feel the same way, however, for me, it drives my choices. When I feel that I am not making a contribution, guilt and regret set in. As a result, I have always maintained a high level of participation in all of the responsibilities around our house. It hasn't been easy.

In the early years, Ellen and I would alternate nights with Jacob, which meant little to no sleep followed by a long day of work. Trimming down a work trip from five to three days so that I could be home meant driving from city to city late at night or early in the morning. Over time, the lack of sleep and constant lifting Jacob up and down stairs took its toll. We were exhausted. There had to be a better way, a smarter way. So we moved Jacob to the main floor of our house, and when Jacob turned 17, we switched our caregiver to work nights so we could sleep. This last move was a game changer. But then I started suffering from back pain.

Whether it was from waterskiing, lifting Jacob or something hereditary, I don't know. All I knew was that for two years I was a mess, and I couldn't be the contributor I wanted—no, needed— to be. That meant pressure on Ellen to do more with Jacob, and emotional pressure on me because I couldn't help by giving my all. When it was my night to be "on" for Jacob, and he coughed, I was physically limited. I couldn't get out of bed and down to him in time for it to make a difference. And if I did, I often couldn't turn him effectively without experiencing excruciating pain. The turning point occurred one morning at around 4 am when Ellen found me writhing on the floor because, after helping Jacob, I couldn't climb the stairs. I was 49, turning 90. Stubbornness and fear lost the battle. I was going in for back surgery. I had no choice. I had effectively lost control of my ability to contribute and, in fact, had become a burden. Both realities were unacceptable.

I learned two important life lessons from this episode. First, it's important to identify health issues early and deal with them right away. My health is way too important, in all aspects of my family life, not to attend to. Second, Ellen and I have gotten very good at working as a team. I know her strengths and she knows mine, and they are different but complementary. We often joke that our "camps" are so rigid, that if I stray into her camp, she lets me know and I do the same. It's when one of us crosses the line because we want to contribute that the messiness appears. Not only has this knowledge helped our marriage in many ways, but it also makes us work efficiently, whether we are going through times of joy or challenge.

So, was this an easy task to write this piece? No. Was it cathartic, did I gain from it? Yes. Am I happy I did it? Yes. Once again, Ellen, thanks. You were right.

Acknowledgments

Before I begin any book, I flip straight to the acknowledgments. I want to know what makes the author tick, where the story came from. I enjoy reading the testament to all of the people who helped along the journey to getting the story on shelves. The acknowledgments are all about showing gratitude, and that's what I feel every day: Grateful.

Thank you to my editor, Randi Chapnik Myers, for pushing me for more and setting challenges each day to help me to find my voice. I will miss our back and forth e-mails and your brutal honesty when I needed it most. Also many thanks to Jonathan Schmidt for your guidance and support during the writing process. Robert Mackwood, thank you for believing in our story and publishing this book because you knew it was written from the heart. Kudos also to Melanie and Marnie, two of my oldest friends. Every time you read through each chapter and declared, "Ellen, I love it!" I got the boost of confidence I needed to continue. Thank you Craig Offman and Nancy Stitt for reading through the entire manuscript and providing your input. Thank you Catherine Leek, Beth Crane, Cynthia Cake and Heidy Lawrance for transforming my manuscript into this book.

Nora Glass and Jessica Palmer and the Jacob's Ladder Board of Directors, thank you for all the dedication and love over the past

16 years. Bert Stitt, I'll never forget the day we approached you with the idea of setting up a charity, and your exact words were: Consider it done! Look how far we have come together!

Thank you to every person who has helped Jacob's Ladder climb to the heights it has reached. We are a close-knit family, built on hard work, volunteerism and community kindness. We appreciate the countless hours and valuable dollars you have donated to help a little charity grow to what it is today, an important cause with massive heart.

To my Project Give Back team, a team made up of angels. Without our Board of Directors and our supportive sponsors we couldn't reach so many children each year. Thank you teachers for pouring everything you have into teaching and inspiring our young students to be their best selves. Your light leads them to their shining moments.

Thank you to the beautiful helpers who inspire Jacob every day. The teachers at Park Lane School and the Beverley School believe in the most fragile people in our world. The love and stimulation you give to Jacob, from 9 until 3 each day, is everything.

Dara Kahane and Bayview Glen Day Camp, thank you for allowing the sun to shine through the clouds on Jakey in the summer months. To all of Jakey's loving counselors over the years – we are forever grateful for your love, friendship, acceptance and patience. You will forever be Jakey's summer angels.

Jacob's caregivers shower him with love and kindness. They take pride in their relationship with him and allow him to have such dignity and composure. A special thanks goes to Melda,

Cecille, Rina and Anne. I don't know what we would do without you in our lives. Thank you to our caring and attentive CCAC coordinator, Sheena Lynn Bugante and the compassionate PACT team at the Hospital for Sick Children, the Temmy Latner Palliative Care Centre and the Norman Saunders Complex Care Initiative.

A heartfelt thank you to Dr. Jeremy Friedman, Dr. Michael Peer and Dr. Shelley Weiss for years of helping us to navigate the medical challenges of Jacob's complex needs. We cherish the guidance, expertise, professionalism and friendship that you continue to demonstrate.

To our friends and family: Wow, how lucky are we? Our friends are like family and our family are like friends. New and old, we treasure you. You give us strength and laughter and we feel so blessed to be included in your world. Thank you for your continuous check-ins by e-mail, phone, text and weekend visits. We can never have enough of you in our lives.

When I think of my Mom and Dad, I get all teary. Early in the book, I quote a doctor who said, "You are only as happy as your unhappiest child." What would he say about a grandparent's love? The uncompromising support of my parents has helped lighten even the heaviest of days. They can tell what we need just from "hello" and they don't stop to think. They just come rushing. Thank you for being our all-star cheerleaders and my "go to" for almost everything.

Bev, Ben and Jacob. Being your mom has been the greatest gift in my life. When you are pregnant, you have nine months to concoct in your mind who this person kicking inside you might be. I could never have dreamed up better people than you three. I love you with everything I have. You are my inspiration, my hope, my joy and my greatest pride.

Jeff, every day that I get to be your wife, I love you more and more. Thank you for bringing out in me a person that I didn't even know existed. Thank you for being my rock, my devil's advocate and my best friend. Who knows where our life will lead, but with you by my side, I know we can tackle anything together.